Springer
Tokyo
Berlin
Heidelberg
New York
Barcelona
Hong Kong
London
Milan
Paris
Singapore

Y. Haruki, I. Homma
A. Umezawa, Y. Masaoka (Eds.)

Respiration and Emotion

With 56 Figures

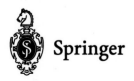 Springer

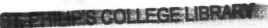

Yutaka Haruki, Ph.D.
School of Human Science
Waseda University
2-579-15 Mikajima, Tokorozawa, Saitama 359-1192, Japan

Ikuo Homma, M.D., Ph.D.
Second Department of Physiology
Showa University School of Medicine
1-5-8 Hatanodai, Shinagawa-ku, Toyko 142-8555, Japan

Akio Umezawa
Department of Psychology
Fukui University
3-9-1 Bunkyo, Fukui 910-8507, Japan

Yuri Masaoka
Second Department of Physiology
Showa University School of Medicine
1-5-8 Hatanodai, Shinagawa-ku, Toyko 142-8555, Japan

ISBN 4-431-70286-5 Springer-Verlag Tokyo Berlin Heidelberg New York

Typesetting: Camera-ready by the editors and authors
Printing and binding: Best-set Typesetter Ltd., Hong Kong
SPIN: 10754245

Preface

Brain research has made progress from technological developments in the field of neuroscience and cognitive neuropsychology; cognition and emotions corresponding to local neuronal activity are revealed scientifically. Emotions are the result of activity within the brain. In addition, their expression always is accompanied by physiological activity such as changes in perspiration, heart rate, and respiration. In other words, emotions are mirrored in physiological responses.

In respiratory physiology, interest in sensation-related respiratory dysfunction has focused on the effect of the higher centers of the brain on respiratory activity. Research on respiratory dysfunctions such as asthma, panic disorder, and hyperventilation syndrome cannot neglect the role of the forebrain and limbic system, however.

This book contains material from the International Interdisciplinary Symposium on Respiration: Respiration and Emotion, held in Tokyo July 23–25, 1999. The aim of the symposium was to present and discuss with people from many countries respiration from many aspects: physiology, psychology, behavioral medicine, and other fields. Not only does the book provide contributions from a scientific approach to respiration, but this research also presents traditional thought regarding breathing as expressed in the Japanese arts. Looking toward the 21st century, research is opening doors to many different fields across all scientific and artistic borders.

We are truly grateful for the support of the Ibuka Fund of Waseda University for this symposium. The symposium required assistance from many people. In particular, we are grateful to Dr. Ishii and Dr. Suzuki for their advice and support. We also thank Ms. Suga, Ms. Kono, and Ms. Takeuchi for their assistance. We are pleased to have had the opportunity to work with Mr. Kenneth Ellis, helping us as an interpreter. The symposium could not have been held without the support of these individuals.

YUTAKA HARUKI
IKUO HOMMA
AKIO UMEZAWA
YURI MASAOKA

Contents

The Art of Breathing in the East and the West

Respiration and Emotion (II)

Special Lecture

Behavioral Breathing and Sensation

Location and Electric Current Sources of Breathlessness in the Human Brain

Ikuo Homma, Arata Kanamaru and Yuri Masaoka

Second Department of Physiology, Showa University School of Medicine, 1-5-8 Hatanodai, Shinagawa-ku, Tokyo 142-8555, Japan

Summary: Breathlessness is an unpleasant sensation associated with breathing and one of the major symptoms in patients with chronic respiratory diseases. There are many sources of breathlessness emphasized by several researchers. However, the localization of the source generator for breathlessness in the human brain has not been made clear. In this study we demonstrated the location of the source generator for breathlessness in humans induced by CO_2 and a resistive load using the dipole tracing method. Five male volunteers participated in this study. The subjects inhaled 5% or 7%CO_2 with a resistive pipe, while EEG and flow were monitored. EEG potentials(20) were triggered to be averaged at the onset of inspiration. A large positive potential wave was observed between 200 to 600msec from the onset of inspiration during 7%CO_2 inhalation with a higher resistive load. The breathlessness rate measured by VAS was high in 7%CO_2 with higher resistive load. The location of the source generator of the large potential, estimated using the SSB-DT method, was found in the limbic system. The results suggest that the source generator for breathlessness, as well as other unpleasant emotional sensations, may be located in the limbic system.

Keyword: dipole tracing method, breathlessness, limbic system, EEG

DIPOLE TRACING METHOD OF THE SCALP-SKULL-BRAIN HEAD MODEL (SSB-DT)

There are a billion neurons in the human brain. Each neuron is polarized and makes a dipole between the synapse and the axon hillock of the cell soma. Depolarization of the membrane under the synapse is referred to as a "sink" of current dipole, and the axon hillock in the cell soma is a "source" of the current. If there is a large number of depolarization in the limited area of the brain, these neurons can be approximated to one or two equivalent current dipoles. From the scalp, potentials of approximately 10μ volts can be recorded from the amount of action potentials. The electric activity in the cerebral cortex can be recorded with surface electrodes mounted on the scalp. The dipole tracing (DT) method estimates the position and the vector dipole moment of an equivalent current dipole from the recorded EEG data[1].

Activities of the brain can be approximated by one or two equivalent current dipoles. Locations of sources and vector moments of the equivalent current dipoles can be estimated from potentials distributed on the scalp and recorded by the surface electrodes. Location of the source is determined by calculating algorithms that minimize the square difference between potentials actually recorded from the scalp (Vmeas) and those calculated from the equivalent dipoles (Vcal). Therefore, locations of the dipoles and vector moments are iteratively changed using the simplex method until the square difference between Vmeas and Vcal becomes minimum. The basic concept of the dipole tracing (DT) method is based on the least square algorithm for fitting the calculated potential to the measured EEG potentials (Fig.1).

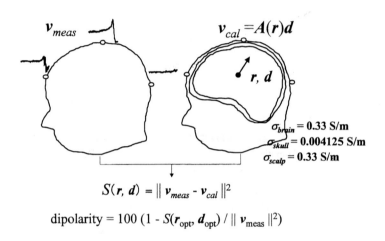

$$S(r, d) = \| v_{meas} - v_{cal} \|^2$$

$$\text{dipolarity} = 100\,(1 - S(r_{opt}, d_{opt}) / \| v_{meas} \|^2)$$

Fig.1. The dipole tracing method: the least square algorithm for fitting the calculated potential. The conductivities of brain (0.33s/m), skull(0.004125s/m) and scalp(0.33s/m) are shown.

Most important thing in estimating the location of the source generator by the DT method is to determine the different conductivities of the scalp, skull and brain. In particular, conductivity of the skull is much smaller than those of the scalp and the brain. It is necessary to reconstruct the shapes of these three layers. Therefore, each subject's own three-layer-head model must be made from CT images[2].

For estimating the location of the source in the brain the following procedure must be used : 1.Record EEG. 2.Measure all electrode positions including reference points (nasion, inion, bilateral pre-meatus points and vertex) with a three-dimensional digitizer. 3.Make each subject's own shape of scalp, skull and brain from CT images. 4.Add different conductivities of the scalp, skull and brain.

The reconstruction of the scalp and the location of the electrode are shown in Fig.2

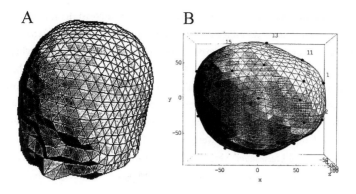

Fig.2. The reconstruction of the scalp(A) and the location of the electrodes on the scalp(B).

DT FOR BREATHLESSNESS

Breathlessness is one of the major symptoms observed not only in chronic respiratory disease but also in many other diseases. Breathlessness is described as an unpleasant sensation associated with respiratory movement. Breathlessness is expressed as 'dyspnea', 'air hunger', 'suffocation', 'chest wall tightness' and others. General sensations such as pain or heat, etc., have their own sensory center and specific receptors. Even though breathlessness is defined as a sensory experience, its sensory receptors have not been specified and the center for breathlessness has not been identified yet. Breathlessness is signals arising from the organism and to know the level of breathlessness is to know the alarming of the body.   In patients with COPD a decrease of breathlessness improves their quality of life. Therefore, it is important to specify the central mechanism in the brain of people with breathlessness.   It is also necessary to clarify the relationship within the structure of the brain and between peripheral receptors and brain activity.

MATERIAL AND METHOD

The study was performed on 5 normal subjects (all males aged 21 to 32) with no history of chronic pulmonary diseases and /or neuromuscular disease. All subjects were naïve to the purpose of the study and signed an informed consent. The subjects breathed through a mouthpiece of a one-way valve with a hotwire flow meter (Minato Ikagaku RF-HE). A resistive pipe (diameter: 6mm or 4mm, length: 100mm) was attached to the inspiratory side of the valve to add load during inspiration. Subjects inhaled 5% or 7% carbon dioxide (CO_2) with oxygen through this valve. During the experiment, the subjects EEG and flow were monitored. A pressure transducer attached to the mouthpiece measured airway pressure. Subjective sensations of breathlessness and hard-to-breathe were measured by the visual analogue scale (VAS) with a line of length of 12cm. Twenty-one electrodes were arranged according to the International 10/20 system over the scalp surface with the reference electrode on the right earlobe to record EEG. EEG was amplified and filtered (band passed:0. 016 to 200Hz, NEC San-Ei 6R 12) and stored on an EEG analyzer (Nihon Kohden DAE-2100). Twenty-one electrode positions and the reference point positions (nasion, inion, bilateral pre-meatus points and vertex) were measured with a three-dimensional digitizer (Science 3DL). After the experiment, CT images of the head were obtained from each subject. Wire-frame models for the shaped scalp, skull and brain layer were reconstructed from the CT images. EEGs of twenty breath cycles of the different CO_2 and resistive pipes were triggered to average from the onset of inspiration. The experimental setting is illustrated in Fig.3

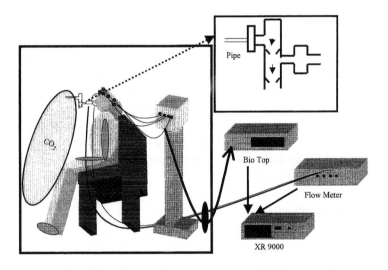

Fig.3. Experimental Design.

RESULTS

Changes of mouth pressure, respiratory rate (RR), tidal volume (VT) and breathlessness (VAS) during inhaling 5% or 7% CO_2 through resistive pipes of 4x100mm or 6x100mm are shown in Table

1. Mean mouth pressure during inspiration with a resistive pipe of 6x100mm was -7.94 ± 3.30 cmH$_2$O during 5% CO_2 inhalation and -7.42 ± 2.42 cmH$_2$O during 7% CO_2 inhalation. Mean mouth pressure with a resistive pipe of 4x100mm was -13.26 ± 4.72 cmH$_2$O during 5% CO_2 inhalation and -13.96 ± 2.86 cmH$_2$O during 7% CO_2 inhalation . Subjective sensation of breathlessness increased during the inhalation of 7% CO_2 and with a higher resistive load. Fig.4 shows averaged 20 EEG triggered at the onset of inspiration in one subject.

Table 1. Mouthpressure(cmH$_2$O), respiratory rate (RR n/min), tidal volume (VT) and breathlessness (VAS) during inhalation of 5% or 7% CO_2 through resistive pipes of 4×100mm and 6×100mm.

		5%		7%	
		4×100	6×100	4×100	6×100
Pressure (cm H$_2$O)		-13.26 ± 4.72	-7.94 ± 3.30	-13.96 ± 2.86	-7.42 ± 2.42
RR (n/min)		16.80 ± 2.48 (C)	15.80 ± 4.41 (C)	15.90 ± 2.79 (C)	15.90 ± 2.79 (C)
		19.10 ± 4.67 (L)	17.45 ± 3.86 (L)	18.05 ± 5.08 (L)	17.10 ± 5.05 (L)
V$_T$ (ml)		544 ± 114 (C)	547 ± 114 (C)	530 ± 99 (C)	530 ± 99 (C)
		1065 ± 202 (L)	1080 ± 212 (L)	1283 ± 193 (L)	1192 ± 178 (L)
VAS	CO$_2$	4.97 ± 1.53	3.92 ± 1.89	6.33 ± 2.65	5.42 ± 2.61
	Resistive Load	7.85 ± 0.79	6.57 ± 1.26	8.33 ± 1.07	6.90 ± 1.95
	Hard to Breath	8.10 ± 0.85	5.57 ± 0.80	8.30 ± 1.36	5.77 ± 2.13

5% CO_2 + 6×100 7% CO_2 + 4×100

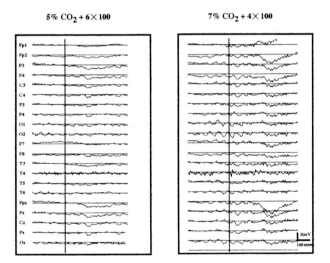

Fig.4. Averaged 20 EEG recordings triggered at the onset of inspiration (vertical lines). Left shows EEG during inhalation of 5%CO2 through a resistive pipe of 6×100mm. Right shows EEG during inhalation of 7%CO2 through a resistive pipe of 4×100mm.

The left side of the figure shows averaged EEG when the subject breathed 5%CO_2 with a lower resistive load. The right shows averaged EEG when the subject breathed 7%CO_2 with a higher resistive load. A large positive potential change was observed between 200msec to 400msec from the onset of inspiration during 7%CO_2 breathing with a high resistive load. These large potential changes were also observed in 4 other subjects. The locations of the equivalent current dipole of this large potential were estimated using the dipole tracing method.

7% 4-100

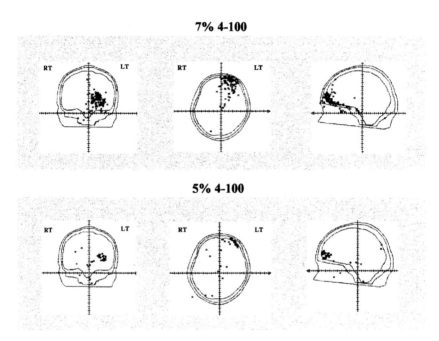

5% 4-100

Fig.5. The locations of dipoles in the brain during 7%CO_2 (upper) and 5%CO_2 (lower) breathing with a resistive pipe of 4×100mm. The left panels show the coronal section view, the middle panels show the axial section view and the right panels show the saggital section views.

The locations of dipoles in the brain during 7%CO_2 and 5%CO_2 breathing with a higher resistive load are shown in Fig.5. The left panels in the figure show the coronal section view, the middle panels show the axial section view and the right panels show the saggital section view. From the estimation of the dipole tracing method, the locations of the source generator were observed in the frontal cortex and in the limbic or Para limbic cortex. Dipolarity, which shows the accuracy of the estimation, was 97%.

DISCUSSION

Recently several non-invasive methods such as positron emission tomography (PET) or functional magnetic resonance imaging (fMRI) have been used to examine the area of the active brain site. Colebatch et al (1991)[3] and Ramsey et al (1993)[4] showed the active area in the brain during volitional breathing in humans. Changes of regional cerebral blood flow examined by PET reflect regional neural activities. Fink et al (1996)[5] also showed the active area in the brain during exercise-induced hyperpnoea using PET. The areas were the bilateral supralateral primary motor cortex and associated motor cortex which Colebatch et al (1991) and Ramsey et al (1993) showed during volitional breathing. Contrary to PET, which indirectly shows neural activities, EEG shows neural activities directly[3,4]. Electrical current recorded by EEG has been thought to be generated in synapses and somas of the neurons. The dipole tracing method estimates the location of dipoles that are generated between synapse and soma. One of the disadvantages of the dipole tracing method is electrical current conductivities in scalp, skull and brain are different. The SSB-DT method has been developed to estimate the location of current dipoles taking into account the differing conductivities[2]. It has been assumed that the location of the spikes in the epileptic patient recorded by subdural electrodes agrees with the location estimated by the SSB-DT method[6]. Using the SSB-DT method, the location of the source generator for voluntary breathing was shown by Kanamaru et al in 1999[7]. During voluntary breathing, the source generator was estimated in the pre-central sulcus and a few cm lateral to the mid line where according to the work of Penfield and Rasmussen (1950), the primary motor cortex for chest wall muscles exist[8]. Corfield et al (1995) showed active areas during CO_2 breathing in awake humans using PET[9]. They showed neural activation within the limbic system and suggested that the area might be important in the sensory response to hypercapnia. In the present study, we demonstrated the location of the source generator in the limbic system during hypercapnia, especially when the subjects' sensed breathlessness. The limbic system may be important for the sensation of breathlessness as for other unpleasant emotional sensations [10].

REFERENCES

1. He B, Musha T, Okamoto Y, Homma S, Nakajima Y, Sato T (1987) Electric dipole tracing in the brain by means of the boundary element method and its accuracy. IEEE Trans. Biomed. Eng., BME-34, 6:406-414
2. Homma S, Musha T, Nakajima Y, Okamoto Y, Blom S, Flink R, Hagbarth K-E, Mostrom U (1994) Location of electric current sources in the human brain estimated by the dipole tracing method of the scalp-skull-brain (SSB) head model. Electroenceph. Clin. Neurohysiol.,91:374-382
3. Colebatch JG, Adams L, Murphy K, Martin AJ, Lammertsma AA (1991) Regional caerebral blood flow during volitional breathing in man. J. Physiol. 443:91-103
4. Ramsay SC, Adams L, Murphy K, Corfield DR, Grootoonk S, Bailey DL, Frackowiak RSJ, Guz

Respiratory sensations may be controlling elements on ventilation but can be affected by personality traits and state changes

Neil S. Cherniack, Marc H. Lavietes, Lana Tiersky, and Benjamin H. Natelson

University of Medicine and Dentistry of New Jersey, New Jersey Medical School, 185 So. Orange Avenue, MSB/C-671, Newark, New Jersey 07103, USA

Summary. The reflex control of breathing can be modified behaviorally by the cortex, which receives information on respiratory movements and is able to alter ventilation by sending signals to the bulbopontine respiratory neurons and to spinal motor neurons. This behavioral control of respiration can interfere with reflex control during speaking and singing for example; but can also assist reflex control by enhancing responses to chemical stimuli and preventing apneas during wakefulness. It is also possible that behavioral control helps adjust ventilation and breathing patterns to minimize work expenditure and maximize gas exchange. Respiratory sensations are affected both by respiratory movements and by changes in chemoreceptor activity. Sensations increase with ventilation, particularly with greater respiratory efforts per breath and also grow as PCO_2 rises. This behavioral control which might act to modify ventilation and breathing patterns to minimize respiratory sensations could help achieve an optimum compromise between ventilation and PCO_2 levels.

However, respiratory sensations may also be affected by personality traits. We could show that the intensity of respiratory sensations differs among individuals and varies with psychological characteristics like anxiety. Hence, the possible optimizing role of dyspnea is imperfect and at times may be detrimental if dyspnea intensifies anxiety and leads to increased respiratory efforts.

Key Words. Respiratory control, optimization, dyspnea, personality traits

The respiratory rhythm arises from the signals of chemical and mechanical receptors impinging on networks of respiratory neurons in the pons and medulla, and produces a fairly stereotyped sequence of breaths. However, this reflex control can be temporarily overridden by voluntarily actions as in breath holding and speech. [1,2] Changes in alertness, emotional factors, and stress can also alter the pattern and level of breathing for even longer periods of time, sometimes interfering with responses to chemical and mechanical stimuli (CO_2 breathing and inspiratory resistive loads). Quite often though, the activity of higher brain centers is helpful enhancing the accuracy and speed of the response of the control system or extending its scope and range of action. For example, apneas and periodic breathing occur during sleep with resulting drops in blood O_2 levels but are uncommon during wakefulness when cortical influences on breathing are greater, and act to eliminate apneas, even though chemosensitivity is higher in the awake state. [3,4] Greater chemosensitivity would be expected to intensify periodicity and apneas but do not because of "wakefulness" drives, i.e., excitatory signals from higher brain centers to respiratory neurons caused by environmental stimuli.

In addition to its ability to modify respiratory output, higher brain centers can sense the magnitude of respiratory movements. Normal individuals can detect and quantify changes in lung volume, and the size of tidal breaths, and ventilation, in large part via information relayed by muscle proprioceptors. [5] Tack et. al. showed that in their estimations, subjects take into account both volume displacements and the force exerted by the respiratory muscles and that there is an age dependent difference. [6] In experiments which required subjects to produce a range of tidal volumes during unencumbered breathing and then reproduce the same volumes while inspiring through graded resistive and elastic loads, the subjects seemed to integrate both pressure and volume signals in their duplicating attempts. Analysis showed that sensation appears to depend on the product of pressure and volume but each raised to a different power.

Other investigators have demonstrated that respiratory sensations during breathing are determined by the product of force, inspiratory time, and frequency with force (measured from the mouth pressure) as the most important determinant. (Eq. 1) [7]

$$(1) \quad S = P^{1.3} \, ti^{0.52} \, f^{0.19}$$

where S = sensation, P = respiratory pressure, f = breathing frequency, ti= inspiratory time.

OPTIMIZATION OF BREATHING

It has been argued for a number of years that ventilation and breathing patterns are adjusted by the respiratory system so as to minimize the work or energy costs of breathing and to maximize the efficiency of gas exchange. [8] This optimization is likely to be most important in the presence of lung disease when abnormal function decreases respiratory muscle efficiency and elevates the energy costs of breathing. For a given motor nerve output the force generated by the respiratory muscles depends on muscle length while the resulting tidal volume depends on the resistive and elastic forces that oppose the movement of air into the lungs produced by the force of muscle contraction. At one time it was believed that respiratory motor nerve output was fixed by the level of arterial PCO_2 and PO_2, i.e. on peripheral and central chemoreceptor activity. However, it was shown that conscious humans faced with an inspiratory load increased their "occlusion pressure", a measure of motor nerve electrical activity, at all levels of chemical drive. [9] Also, the observation that patterns of breathing tend to be different depending upon whether the forces opposing air movement are elastic or resistive suggested that criteria other than were considered by the respiratory controller in setting the size of tidal volume. [10] To the present time, no receptors capable of responding to differences in work level (ergoreceptors) have been found. Thus the idea that work was optimized was replaced by the idea that humans minimized respiratory pressure swings. [11]

Poon proposed that breathing levels and not just breathing patterns were optimized and were set to maximize a figure of merit, which depended both on ventilation and chemical drive and prevented either from becoming too great. [12] This is shown in equation 2.

$$(2) \; J = 2 \ln V + a \, (PCO_2 - B)^2$$

when J = figure of merit, PCO_2 = arterial PCO_2, and V = ventilation

Because respiratory sensations depend both on volume and muscle force, it seemed possible that the cortex in order to minimize awareness of respiratory sensations might also act at least roughly to minimize breathing work particularly when there was some prolonged impediment to breathing. Acutely, subjects faced with breathing impediments seemed to try to overcome them, magnifying the output of the respiratory muscles and increasing temporarily respiratory work. [8,9]

13

We have shown in the past that large voluntary variations in breathing from the usual level either up or down increase awareness of breathing, i.e. "dyspnea" in normal subjects. [12] Sensations of dyspnea also heighten with increased chemical drive, so that if ventilation is kept constant, dyspnea increases as PCO_2 levels rise. [13,14] Although dyspnea occurs with increased respiratory work or effort, greater ventilation lowers chemical drives. Thus, dyspnea could act as an optimizing principle adjusting drives to breathe so that awareness is reduced and thereby serving to help minimize respiratory work as well. A mathematical model which describes changes in respiratory sensations with rising PCO_2 with ventilation determined by reflex action (automatic control) and with voluntary control has been constructed by Oku. [15] and is shown diagrammatically in Figure 1.

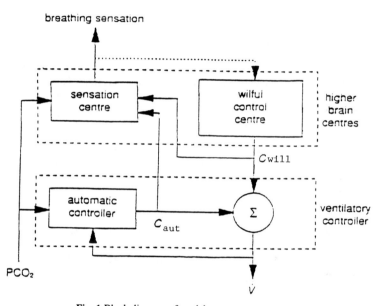

Fig. 1 Block diagram of model

In the model, ventilation depends on the sum of the activity of an automatic controller, which is sensitive to changes in PCO_2 and is inhibited by ventilation changes (an inhibitory neuromechanical feed back) and on the activity of a willful controller, which allows ventilation to be voluntarily changed.

Signals proportional to the motor commands of the automatic and of the willful motor controllers and a signal proportional to PCO_2 are transmitted to a sensation center so that sensation (S) varies according to the following equation 3.

$$(3) \quad S = C^2 aut + K_0 C^2 will + K_1 (PCO_2 - P_0)^2$$

where S = sensation, Caut = the output of the reflex (automatic) control system, Cwill = voluntary motor output, and PCO_2 = arterial PCO_2

Cwill can be either positive or negative since willful commands can either decrease or increase ventilation.

The results are consistent with experiments that show CO_2 can act independently of ventilation to increase respiratory sensations and that voluntary restraint of ventilation amplifies sensations more than does voluntary over breathing. [13]

Like Poon's equation, the equation describing sensation changes varies both with PCO_2 and with ventilation. [12,15,16] Thus, the model supports the idea that the sense of dyspnea could act as an optimizing factor by enhancing a figure of merit like the one proposed by Poon. Note that in the model all increases in respiratory sensations are treated the same whatever their quality of unpleasantness. Thus the model ignores the differences in the terms that have used to describe sensations. [17,18]

EMOTIONAL STATUS & DYSPNEA

While dyspnea could serve an optimizing role in setting both the level and pattern of breathing, a number of different factors may modify the sensations caused by breathing leading to considerable inter-individual variability in the intensity of dyspnea produced by a given increment in respiratory work or effort. These factors include age and experience with changed respiratory muscle mechanics, but personality traits may be especially important. [18,19,20]

We carried out the following studies to see how personality might affect the sense of dyspnea produced by breathing on inspiratory resistive loads. We were particularly interested in examining the response of subjects who might be expected to amplify symptoms by exaggerating signals arising from physiological or pathophysiological processes.

PROTOCOL FOR EXAMINING PERSONALITY TRAITS

We studied the responses of 2 groups of subjects (free from organic disease) to two levels of inspiratory resistive loading: a group of 29 subjects with well-defined chronic fatigue syndrome (CFS); and another group of 23, age and gender matched controls. We chose CFS subjects because symptom amplification is thought to explain, in part, the symptoms of CFS. [21,22] We used the Borg scale to obtain their estimates of the magnitude of dyspnea experienced during loading [23]. Measurements of ventilation served as measures of their objective responses to loading. Each subject received an extensive psychological assessment as subsequently described.

Screening pulmonary function tests, which included the vital capacity and forced expiratory volume in one second were performed with a standard spirometric system. Subjects sat in a comfortable chair, arms supported by arm rests. They inspired through a mouthpiece, wearing nose clips, from an open circuit. End-tidal CO_2 was sampled continuously from the mouthpiece. Throughout the loaded breathing trials, inspiratory flow was measured with a pneumotachygraph.

The modified Borg scale was used to assess dyspnea throughout the loaded breathing trials. [23] Subjects were asked to scale "discomfort with breathing". Subjects were asked to think of zero as "no discomfort whatsoever" and ten as "the most discomfort you have ever associated with breathing". Subjects were to grade their sense of dyspnea at various intervals throughout the protocol.

Subjects also underwent a clinical psychiatric interview using the Quick Diagnostic Interview Schedule (Q-DIS). [24,25] Both standardized tests of depressive symptoms (the Center of Epidemiological Study depression scale, or CESD) and the Neuroticism subscale of the NEO Personality Inventory-Revised (NEO PI-R) were administered. [23,24] Subjects were also asked whether or not they had ever been given a standard psychiatric diagnosis as defined by the DSM-III.

Subjects assessed their degree of discomfort before breathing on the mouthpiece, while breathing quietly through the mouthpiece until air flow and end-tidal PCO_2 tracings were stable, and again 30 seconds after a small resistive load (1.34 cm $H_2O/l/s$ measured at 1.0 l/s) had been surreptitiously added to the inspiratory side of the breathing circuit. A final estimate of discomfort was given after the fifth minute. After a brief rest period, these same subjects repeated the entire protocol; this time, a larger load (3.54 cm $H_2O/l/s$ measured at 1.0 l/s) was used. For the 27 subjects who participated in the entire protocol, measurements of minute ventilation (V) were made at the following intervals: 20s, 40s, one minute, 90s, and 2, 3, 4, and 5 minutes. The experimenters performing the tests and analyzing the data did not know which subjects belonged to the CFS or non-CFS groups. Data analysis was performed with a standard statistical package.

In addition to comparing data from CFS and non-CFS subjects, we also identified "responders" and "non-responders" in both groups. Among the 52 subjects, 23 reported a higher Borg score within 30s after introduction of the small load; these subjects were defined as "responders". The other 29, who did not report an increased Borg score after introduction of the small load were called "non-responders". Of the 27 subjects who participated in the extended loading protocol, 10 were responders; 17, non-responders. CFS subjects were distributed evenly between the "responders" and "non-responders".

RESPONSES OF CHRONIC FATIGUE SYNDROME PATIENTS

For CFS subjects, the mean Borg score prior to introduction of the small load was 1.24 Borg scale units; for the non-CFS, 1.04. Immediately after loading, the mean Borg response for the CFS group rose to 1.71, and for the non-CFS group to 1.67. These differences were not statistically significant. Neither group reported a statistically significant increase in Borg response following the addition of the smaller load. V for CFS subjects prior to loading, 12.9 ± 0.65 (SEM), did not differ from that of the non-CFS group, 11.4 ± 3.9. There was no change in ventilation seen in either group immediately following loading.

However, differences were found between groups with respect to their psychological profile. CFS subjects scored 76 ± 33 (SD) on the neuroticism scale; non-CFS, 54 ± 19 (t = 2.83; p = < .007). Similarly, CFS subjects scored higher on the CESD depression scale (22 ± 14 SD) than did non-CFS subjects (5 ± 4; t = 6.35. p≤0.001).

RESPONDERS VS. NON-RESPONDERS

There were no differences between "responders" vs. "non-responders" with respect to age, height, weight, and lung function. V and Borg scores for both the "responder" and "non-responder" group subjects who participated in the extended protocol are as follows.

There was no significant difference between V prior to the introduction of the small load which was 13.3 ± 3.6 (SD) l/m in the R group; and the V of 12.5 ± 4.6 in the NR group. In the responder group Borg scores increased with loading, but not in the non-responders. Ventilation was higher initially and remained higher in the responders vs. the non-responders on the smaller load.

In both groups Borg scores were higher on the larger than on the smaller load. There were no significant differences in V in the two groups over the 5 minutes of breathing on the larger resistive load. However, he Borg score increased progressively over time for the R, but not the NR group on the larger load. Statistical analysis showed significant differences between the means of the groups for all Borg data for both the larger and smaller load when compared at different time intervals during loaded breathing. Data on the Borg scores for the larger load are shown in Figure 2.

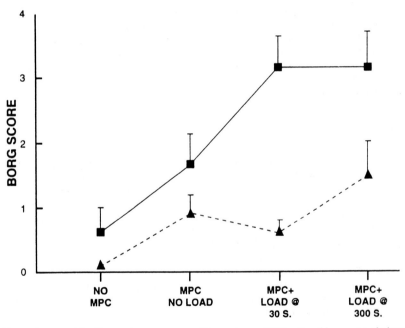

Fig. 2 ▲--------- Non-Responders ■——— Responders   MPC = Breathing on mouthpiece
Borg scores obtained while breathing on the larger resistive load

Individual data showed some overlap between groups, however. For example, Borg scores given by R subjects 30 seconds following the introduction of the large load ranged from 3 to 9; while for the 13 NR subjects, from zero to 5. Inspiratory flow, inspiratory time and tidal volume during loaded breathing were not different in R and NR groups on the larger load.

Complete data for psychological testing was available for 46 subjects. There was a positive correlation between the Borg score selected by each subject during mouthpiece breathing but before introduction of the load and his score on the neuroticism measure (p=0.029; Spearman's rank correlation test). A higher prevalence of psychopathology was found in the R group. Specifically, 45% of the R group subjects met the DSM III-R diagnostic criteria for a psychiatric disorder, whereas only 17% of the non-responder subjects met such criteria. The R group subjects had higher depression scores than did NR subjects (t=2.04; p=0.049). The CESD score for CFS subjects in the responder group (30 ± 14 SD) was greater than the CESD score for the CFS subjects in the non-responder group (15 ± 10; t = 2.65; p < 0.02). By contrast, there was no difference between the CESD scores of the non-CFS subjects in the R and NR groups.

INTERPRETATION

This study suggests that there are subsets of individuals who consistently report more discomfort when presented with inspiratory loads. Individuals who experienced more discomfort on a relatively small load also reported more discomfort on a larger load. The fact that the responses of our two groups remained clearly separated while breathing through the larger load though their ventilation and breathing patterns were nearly the same suggests that the introduction of an easily perceived load may be an appropriate tool for the general study of personality effects and symptom amplification on respiration.

Many stimuli, which have been used previously to study symptom amplification, elicit both physiologic and sensory responses. Submersion of an extremity in ice water, for example, elicits both a physiological response (e.g., vasoconstriction, and tachycardia) and a perceptual response, pain. It has however been difficult to separate the intensity of the subjective response from the intensity of the physiological response because those who experience more vasoconstriction have more pain. [25] On the other hand, in our study, both responders and non-responders breathed the same when acutely challenged by the 3.54 cmH$_2$O/l/s load. Psychological characteristics are also likely to affect respiratory sensations when lung function is chronically impaired but the precise effects of particular traits on both the acute and the chronic sensory response remain to be determined.

Psychological factors might increase or decrease an individual's load response. Subjects with the appropriate psychological makeup may symptom amplify, or exhibit an exaggerated subjective response. The symptom amplifier tends to be anxious, self-conscious and have low self-esteem and to report symptoms involving several systems. [25,26] On the other hand, subjects with certain psychological characteristics, e.g "defensiveness", may have a diminished response. [27]

In our study, the "responder" group, demonstrated more depressive symptoms and were more likely to meet the diagnostic criteria for a DSM III-R psychiatric diagnosis than did "non-responder" group subjects. The subset of R group patients who had CFS scored highly on the CESD depression scale. A CESD score of ≥27 is thought to identify subjects with depression. Neuroticism scores differed greatly between CFS and non-CFS subjects while dyspnea scores did not. It is of interest while neuroticism scores were related to Borg scores prior to loading, they were not significantly different in R and NR groups.

CONCLUSIONS

Intense sensations produced by impediments to respiratory movements can lead initially to increased effort to overcome them, but in the long run are distracting, limit activity and lead to strategies to diminish awareness of respiratory sensations. In the end, these strategies may become automatic [3]. Increased respiratory effort or work as well as increased chemical drives to breathe all heighten respiratory sensation. Hence, strategies to diminish sensations would lead also to some compromise between the conflicting goals of low respiratory work and diminished chemical drives.

There are problems in the use of respiratory sensations in optimization. Their intensity only roughly approximates respiratory work or chemical drives so that they do not very accurately mirror changes in either by themselves. However, because respiratory work is fairly low and normally does not have a sharply defined minimum even in lung disease, optimization attempts may not need to be very exact. [29]

Perhaps an even more important limitation is that the intensity of respiratory sensations is modified substantially by personality and by stress. Our data, in fact, show that depression, for example, alters respiratory sensation.

It is possible that particular personality traits may affect specific components of the breathing cycle such as tidal volume or frequency or inspiratory time. [19] For example, a decrease in expiratory time by anxiety could lead to lung overinflation in patients with airway obstruction. [18] An increase in breathing frequency can produce on an overall increase in ventilation which can heighten dyspnea. Panic attacks for example can intensify the breathless produced by episode of bronchoconstriction.

Finally, certain personality traits may obscure the ability to recognize and quantify impediments to breathing as occur in asthma so that the respiratory control system response to dangerous events is delayed or attenuated. [30-32]

1. Orem J and Netick A (1986) Behavioral control of breathing in the cat. Brain Res 366:238-253
2. Sears TA (1971) Breathing: a sensori-motor act. Sci Basis Med Ann Rev 128-147
3. Khoo MCK (1999) Periodic breathing and central apnea. In: Altose MD, Kawakami Y (eds) Control of breathing in health and disease. Marcel Dekker Inc, New York, pp 203-240
4. Cummin AR, Sidhu VS, Telford RJ, Saunders KB (1992) Ventilatory responsiveness to carbon dioxide below the normal control point in conscious normoxic humans. Eur Resp J 5:512-516
5. Wolkove N, Altose MD, Kelsen SG, Kondapalli PG, Cherniack NS (1981) Perception of changes in breathing in normal human subjects. J Appl Physiol 50:78-83
6. Tack M, Altose MD, Cherniack NS (1983) Effects of aging on sensation of respiratory force and displacement. J Appl Physiol 55:1433-1440
7. Killian KJ, Bucens DD, Campbell EJ (1982) Effect of breathing patterns on the perceived magnitude of added loads to breathing. J Appl Physiol 52:578-584
8. Cherniack NS (1996) Respiratory sensation as a respiratory controller. In Adams L, Guz A (eds) Respiratory sensation. Marcel Dekker Inc., New York, pp 213-230
9. Altose MD, McCauley WC, Kelsen SG, Cherniack NS (1977) Effects of hypercapnia and inspiratory flow-resistive loading on respiratory activity in chronic airways obstruction. J Clin Invest 59:500-507
10. Otis AB (1958) The work of breathing. Physiol Rev 34:449-458
11. Mead J (1960) Control of respiratory frequency. J Appl Physiol 15:325-336

12. Poon CS (1987) Ventilatory control in hypercapnia and exercise: optimization hypothesis. J Appl Physiol 62:2441-2459
13. Chonan T, Mulholland MB, Leitner J, Altose MD, Cherniack NS (1990) Sensation of dyspnea during hypercapnia, exercise, and voluntary hyperventilation. J Appl Physiol 68:2100-2106
14. Oku Y, Saidel GM, Cherniack NS, Altose MD (1996) Effects of willful ventilatory control on respiratory sensation during hypercapnia. Resp 63:137-143
15. Oku Y, Saidel GM, Cherniack NS, Altose MD (1995) Model of respiratory sensation and willful control of ventilation. Med Biol Eng and Comput 33:252-256
16. Oku Y, Saidel GM, Altose MD, Cherniack NS (1993) Perceptual contributions to optimization of breathing. Ann Biomed Eng 21:509-515
17. Adams L, Lane R, Shea SA, Cockcroft A, Guz A (1985) Breathlessness during different forms of ventilatory stimulation: a study of mechanisms in normal subjects and respiratory patients. Clin Sci 69:663-672
18. Banzett RB, Lansing RW, Brown R, Topulos GP, Yager D, Steele SM, Londono B, Loring SH, Reid MB, Adams L, et al (1990) "Air hunger" from increased PCO_2 persists after complete neuromuscular block in humans. Resp Physiol 81:1-17
19. Masaoka Y, Homma I (1997) Anxiety and respiratory patterns: their relationship during mental stress and physical load. Int J of Psychophysiol 27:153-159
20. Boiten FA, Frijda NH, Wientjes CJ (1999) Emotions and respiratory patterns: review and critical analysis. Int J Psychophysiol 17:103-128
21. Schluederberg A, Straus SE, Peterson P, Blumenthal S, Komaroff AL, Spring B, Landay A, Buchwald D (1992) Chronic fatigue syndrome research, definition and medical outcome assessment. Ann Int Med 117:325-331
22. Rosen SD, King JC, Wilkinson JB, Nixon PG (1990) Is chronic fatigue syndrome synonymous with effort syndrome? J Royal Soc Med 83:761-764
23. Borg GA (1982) Psychophysical bases of perceived exertion. Med Sci Sports Exercise 14:377-381
24. Radloff LS (1977) The CES-D: a self-report depression scale for research in the general population. Appl Psych Measurement 1:385-401
25. Costa PT Jr, McCrae RR (1992) Revised NEO personality inventory (NEO-P1-R). Professional manual psychological assessment resources. Odessa, FL
26. Gramling SE, Clawson EP, McDonald MK (1996) Perceptual and cognitive abnormality model of hypochondriasis amplification and physiological reactivity in women. Psychosom Med 58:423-431
27. Costa PT Jr, McCrae RR (1980) Somatic complaints in males as a function of age and neuroticism: a longitudinal analysis. J Behavioral Med 3:245-257
28. Isenberg S, Lehrer P, Hochron S (1998) Defensiveness and perception of external inspiratory resistive loads in asthma. J Behavioral Med 20:461-472
29. Yamashiro SM, Daubenspeck JA, Lavritsen TN, Grodins FS (1975) Total work rate optimization in CO_2 inhalation and exercise. J Appl Physiol 38:702-709
30. Rushford N, Tiller JW, Pain MC (1998) Perception of natural fluctuations in peak flow in asthma: clinical severity and psychological correlates. J Asthma 35:251-259
31. Tiller J, Pain MC, Biddle N (1987) Anxiety disorder and perception of inspiratory resistive loads. Chest 91:547-551
32. Priel B, Heimer D, Rabinowitz B, Hendler N (1994) Perceptions of asthma severity: the role of negative affectivity. J Asthma 31:479-484

Respiratory Sensations and the Behavioral Control of Breathing

Steven A Shea

Harvard Medical School, and Circadian, Neuroendocrine & Sleep Disorders Section, Brigham & Women's Hospital, 221 Longwood Avenue, Boston, MA 02115, USA

Summary: Humans can perceive a wide range of respiratory sensations—motion, position, irritation, and generalized feelings including respiratory discomfort. In addition, peripheral and central chemoreceptors' afferents may be perceived and it is believed that information related to the magnitude of respiratory drive is sent to sensory areas of the cortex where they are perceived ('corollary discharge'). Many of these afferent pathways can contribute to the constellation of sensations that comprise clinical reports of dyspnea. In studying these mechanisms, the situation is further complicated by the fact that breathing can be reflexly controlled and voluntarily controlled, and the sensations may be different depending on the source of the motor command to breathe. Our experiments have been designed to examine the basic mechanisms of one specific respiratory sensation: the 'urge to breathe' or 'air hunger' that accompanies derangements in arterial blood gases, exercise and breath-hold. We have documented robust relationships between three interacting variables: the level of ventilation, the level of respiratory drive (induced during hypercapnia or exercise) and the level of the sensation of 'air hunger'. We found that mild hypercapnia induces air hunger; increases in ventilation help relieve this sensation; this relief can be provided by pulmonary stretch receptors; and that people adapt to the prevailing level of arterial carbon dioxide. We also found that the level of ventilation needed to alleviate air hunger during induced hypercapnia is less than the level of spontaneous ventilation. This suggests that spontaneous breathing during blood gas derangement is not behaviorally controlled to minimize discomfort. All of our studies are consistent with the hypothesis that air hunger is caused by a parallel copy of increased brainstem respiratory motor activity ('corollary discharge').

Key words: Respiratory Sensations, Dyspnea, Air Hunger, Ventilation, Behavioral Control.

INTRODUCTION

Humans can perceive a wide range of respiratory sensations—motion, position, irritation, and generalized feelings including respiratory discomfort. In addition, peripheral and central chemoreceptors' afferents may be perceived and it is believed that information related to the magnitude of respiratory drive is sent to sensory areas of the cortex where they are perceived ('corollary discharge'). Many of these afferent pathways can contribute to the constellation of sensations that comprise clinical reports of dyspnea. In studying these mechanisms, the situation is further complicated by the fact that breathing can be reflexly controlled and voluntarily controlled, and the sensations may be different depending on the source of the motor command to breathe [1]. In addition, there is interaction between these variables such that the level of breathing affects the level of respiratory sensations, and respiratory sensations themselves can affect the level of breathing (possibly via the voluntary respiratory control pathway) [1]. This interaction and the neural pathways underlying some sensations of respiratory discomfort are shown schematically in Fig. 1.

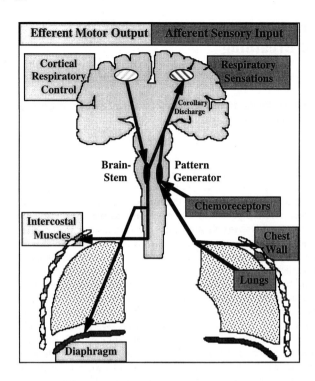

Fig. 1. A simplified diagram of the principal efferent (left) and afferent (right) respiratory control pathways, highlighting the neural pathways underlying some respiratory sensations. A section through the brain, brainstem and spinal cord is shown, along with peripheral respiratory structures.

Our experimental approaches. In order to understand the relationships between breathing and sensation in the face of the complexities of the efferent and afferent control system connections, our studies have concentrated on quantifying one identifiable respiratory sensation namely 'air hunger' or 'shortness of breath'. We have studied this sensation under strictly controlled experimental conditions (controlled levels of mechanical ventilation and blood gases) and during presumed reflex control of breathing (spontaneous breathing during hypercapnia or exercise), as well as overt voluntary control of breathing (breath-hold, speech, voluntary control of mechanical ventilation). We have studied healthy subjects as well as patients with specific neural lesions (high level-quadriplegia, and congenital central hypoventilation syndrome) who enable us to determine the contribution of specific neural pathways to the sensation of air hunger.

Fig. 2. Experimental set-up used in some of our experiments. Subjects were mechanically ventilated, had their blood gases adjusted via control of inspired gases, and reported sensations of air hunger on a 7-point scale. In some experiments the subject was given control of the ventilator via the "Desired Ventilation" controls.

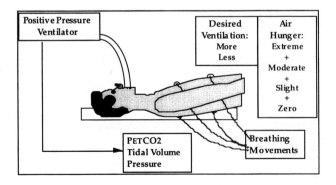

The effect of hypercapnia on air hunger at constant ventilation. Using the set-up shown in Fig. 2, we have previously demonstrated that when the level of ventilation is held constant, healthy subjects begin to perceive air hunger (labeled SLIGHT on the scale, Fig. 2) when end-tidal carbon dioxide (PETCO2) increases by only 3-7 mm Hg above their normal eucapnic level. These healthy subjects felt intolerable air hunger (labeled EXTREME on the scale) when PETCO2 was increased by only 10 mmHg. The most common descriptors of this carbon dioxide induced sensation were "urge to breathe", "like suffocation", "starved for air" and "air hunger" [2]. However, in contrast to fixed mechanical ventilation, these subjects could tolerate higher levels of PETCO2 when breathing spontaneously (at higher levels of ventilation), suggesting that the action of breathing or increased ventilation produces relief of this sensation.

The effect of ventilation on air hunger at a constant level of mild hypercapnia. It is clear that the act of breathing diminishes the air hunger evoked by altered blood gases, as demonstrated by the relief of the discomfort of breath hold by rebreathing alveolar air even though blood gases worsen. In addition, a number of studies have shown that voluntarily reducing breathing below the spontaneous level at a given PETCO2 produces discomfort [1]. In our studies, we found that the sensation of air hunger could be relieved when the experimenter increased the level of mechanical ventilation, and conversely, the sensation of air hunger could be induced or worsened when the experimenter decreased the level of mechanical ventilation. One surprising finding in our studies was that the change in air hunger was not usually immediate after a step change in ventilator tidal volume, despite the likelihood that some afferent neural traffic from the respiratory apparatus would change immediately. Indeed, sometimes the change in sensation took up to 3 minutes to stabilize at a new level following either a step increase or a step decrease in ventilator tidal volume [3]. These studies indicate that the level of ventilation is indirectly proportional to the level of air hunger in the steady-state, but that dynamically there are lags in the system that subserves the reporting of respiratory discomfort. The inertia of sensation to step changes in ventilator tidal volume are shown during mild hypercapnia in Fig. 3.

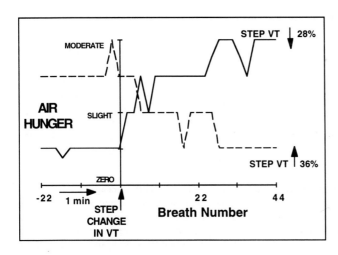

Fig. 3. Effect of a step decrease in ventilator tidal volume (solid line) and a step increase in ventilator tidal volume (dashed line) on air hunger sensation during experimentally induced mild constant hypercapnia ($\approx$ 46 mm Hg) in healthy volunteer subjects. Data derived from Reference [3].

Several neural mechanisms, which are not mutually exclusive, could explain the relief of air hunger provided by breathing: (i) tidal expansion of the lungs and chest, sensed by mechanoreceptors of the lungs, respiratory muscles, and rib joints; (ii) contraction of respiratory pump muscles, as

24

sensed by spindle and tendon organ receptors; (iii) release of the cortical effort needed to inhibit medullary respiratory centers (e.g., as at the end of breath holding); and (iv) flow, sensed by receptors in the upper airways [1]. Voluntarily over-breathing can cause some aspects of respiratory discomfort such as effort, but probably does not increase the urge to breathe. To begin to distinguish among these mechanisms, we further explored the relationship between ventilation and air hunger at a constant level of mild hypercapnia in tetraplegic patients who had high cervical spinal injuries such that they were ventilator-dependent and lacked chest wall afferent information, but had preserved central connections with the vagal afferents from the lungs. Again, increasing ventilation (increased pulmonary stretch receptor activation in absence of changes in blood gases) reduced air hunger showing that vagal afferents (likely pulmonary stretch receptors) alone can provide this relief [4]. An example of one trial in which ventilator tidal volume is adjusted and the tetraplegic subject reports air hunger ratings is shown in Fig. 4.

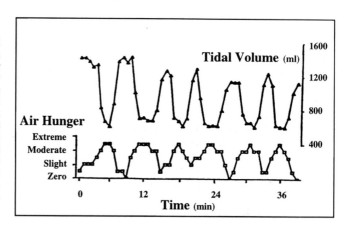

Fig. 4. Altered tidal inflation alters carbon dioxide induced air hunger in a mechanically ventilated tetraplegic patient in whom central connections between chest wall afferent information and the brainstem are severed, but central connections with the vagal afferents from the lungs are preserved. Data derived from Reference [3].

These ventilated patients were chronically hypocapnic because of habitually high levels of mechanical ventilation (this is characteristic of many chronically ventilated patients for unknown reasons, but clearly the ventilation level is not selected to maintain normal arterial carbon dioxide [PaCO2]). We determined whether or not these chronically hypocapnic patients adapt to the prevailing chronic level of PaCO2 [5]. We found that increasing the level of inspired and PaCO2 over a number of days (by adding carbon dioxide to the ventilator circuit) resulted in a subjective tolerance to higher levels of experimentally induced hypercapnia. This study indicates that the level of PaCO2 is directly proportional to the level of air hunger in the steady-state, but that the threshold for this relationship can adapt over a number of days.

The effect of air hunger on ventilation at a constant level of mild hypercapnia. In most situations our uncertainty of the source of the respiratory motor command and the fact that breathing and sensation are mutually interactive presents difficulties in quantitatively assessing the effect of respiratory sensation upon breathing. To better define this relationship, one of our experimental approaches has been to induce mild hypercapnia and then allow subjects to control the level of ventilation voluntarily, based on a pre-determined target level of air hunger. In experiments that are analogous to the stimulus-response relationship between hypercapnia and air hunger at a constant level of mechanical ventilation (see above), we studied the quantitative stimulus-response relationship between air hunger and (subject-controlled) ventilation at a constant level of mild hypercapnia [6]. Subjects controlled the ventilator tidal volume to achieve sensations of zero, slight, or moderate air hunger. The results show a robust inverse relationship between level of ventilation and level of air hunger (as also occurred in the above experiments during experimenter-controlled ventilation).

In additional studies, we compared the ventilatory response to hypercapnia when the subject breathed spontaneously to the response when the subject used forebrain commands to control ventilation—on the basis of minimizing air hunger (achieved with subject-controlled mechanical ventilation) [7]. We found that the spontaneous ventilation in healthy adults during mild hypercapnia significantly exceeded the level of (mechanical) ventilation needed to alleviate air hunger. This suggests that spontaneous breathing is not behaviorally controlled to minimize discomfort, or that mechanical ventilation confers an additional relief of air hunger beyond that provided by spontaneous breathing. Typical results form one subject are shown in Fig. 5.

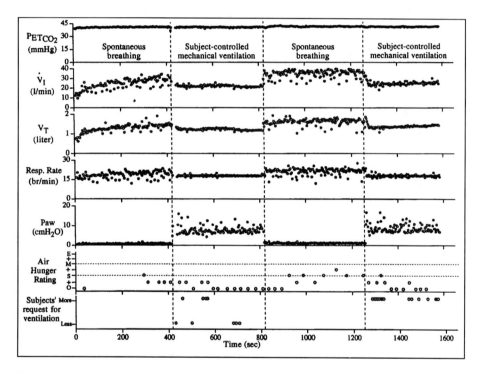

Fig. 5. The level of mechanical ventilation selected by a subject on the basis of minimizing sensations of air hunger is less than the level of spontaneous breathing at equivalent levels of mild induced hypercapnia. Data derived from Reference [7].

The effect of corollary discharge of ventilatory drive on breathing. Patients with Congenital Central Hypoventilation Syndrome (CCHS) lack a ventilatory response to hypercapnia and hypoxia, suggesting a lesion of a common peripheral and central chemoreceptor afferent pathway. Consequently, CCHS patients dangerously hypoventilate during sleep and require assisted ventilation. Nonetheless, many CCHS children can exist quite normally during wakefulness without assisted ventilation, whereby breathing appears to be stimulated by behavioral and arousal related influences [1]. The study of respiratory sensations in CCHS patients provides an opportunity to help determine the neural mechanisms that are responsible for these sensations. For example, if CCHS children experience air hunger during hypercapnia but do not increase breathing, this would disprove the hypothesis that air hunger is caused by a parallel copy of increased brainstem respiratory motor activity ('corollary discharge'). In contrast, if CCHS patients have normal increases in breathing during exercise but do not experience air hunger, this would also disprove the corollary discharge hypothesis. Our results indicate that CCHS patients do not experience respiratory discomfort during induced hypercapnia or during maximal breath hold [8]. The results during exercise were more ambiguous, because at the highest levels of exercise achieved (involving significant anaerobiosis), CCHS subjects reported little respiratory discomfort (less than controls), but they also did not breathe as much as controls during this exercise induced lactic acidosis [8, 9]. Thus, we were unable to disprove the hypothesis that air hunger arises from a projection of corollary discharge to the forebrain [8, 9]. An example of the ventilatory and sensation response to intense exercise above the anaerobic threshold is shown from data in a typical CCHS patient in Fig. 6.

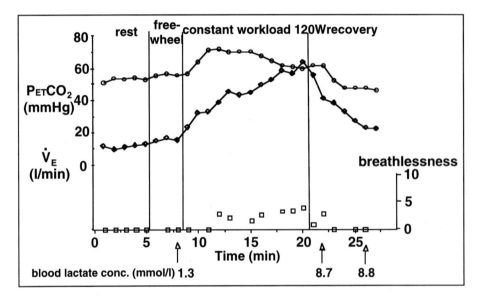

Fig. 6. A patient with CCHS increases breathing during exercise, and at the end of exercise begins to report breathlessness (akin to 'air hunger'). The level of ventilation and the level of breathlessness are both less in CCHS patients than in controls during heavy exercise [8, 9]. These results are consistent with the corollary discharge hypothesis of air hunger. Data derived from Reference [9].

Interaction between reflex and behavioral control of breathing during carbon dioxide induced air hunger. Speech provides a good example of the competition between the behavioral and automatic respiratory control systems. The flow requirements for normal speech exceed resting ventilation, and so subjects hyperventilate when they speak at rest. However, as the automatic drive is increased, say by exercise, the subject will have some control of whether to maintain their speech quality at the expense of reduced breathing, or to increase the airflow during speech (thereby altering speech quality) to maintain their gas exchange. Nevertheless, in this situation, the air used for speech has already been used for gas exchange, so the behavioral and automatic respiratory drives are not completely mutually exclusive. We investigated a novel situation of complete antagonism between the airflow requirements for speech and gas exchange by studying ventilator-dependent tracheotomized subjects who can 'steal' air from alveolar ventilation during the ventilator's inflation phase to produce sound [10]. Thus, speech produced relative hypoventilation and hypercapnia. An example in one subject is shown in Fig. 7.

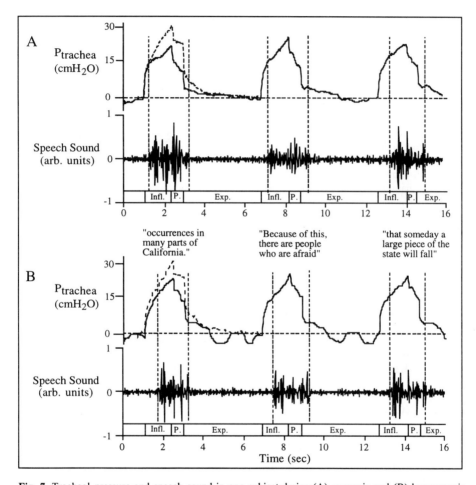

Fig. 7. Tracheal pressure and speech sound in one subject during (A) eucapnia and (B) hypercapnia. The beginning and end of speech for each breath is indicated by dashed vertical lines. In this example, the subject was saying the same phrases on the corresponding breaths during the eucapnic and hypercapnic sequences, as indicated by the text in the center. The ventilator phases are shown (Infl. = inflation; P. = pause at end inflation; Exp. = expiration). The dashed waveform superimposed on the first breath in each condition represents the passive inflation pressure without speech. Note, the loss of air to speech during inflation is indicated by the reduced inflation pressure when speaking. This subject was attempting to supplement the ventilator tidal volume during hypercapnia, as indicated by the substantial phasic inspiratory muscle activity seen on the tracheal pressure waveform throughout the expiratory portion of the ventilator cycle. Data derived from Reference [10].

During induced hypercapnia sufficient to cause significant air hunger, we found that all subjects could still speak adequately. Some subjects 'adapted' by reducing the air used for speech during inflation. In contrast, other subjects reacted as normal subjects do during hypercapnic speech, by increasing the airflow per syllable (a mal-adaptive strategy in ventilated subjects, because this causes greater hypoventilation). These adaptive or mal-adaptive changes were modest despite the strong hypercapnic stimulus. No subject adapted fully, by consistently not speaking on the ventilator's inflation phase. We concluded that modest air hunger modified but never fully suppressed the ability to behaviorally control breathing for purposes of speech [10].

CONCLUSIONS

Our experiments show robust relationships between three interacting variables: the level of ventilation, the level of respiratory drive (induced during hypercapnia or exercise) and the level of the sensation of an 'urge to breathe' or 'air hunger'. We found that mild hypercapnia induces air hunger; increases in ventilation help relieve this sensation; this relief can be provided by pulmonary stretch receptors; and people adapt to the prevailing level of arterial carbon dioxide. We also found that the level of ventilation needed to alleviate air hunger is less than the level of spontaneous ventilation, suggesting that spontaneous breathing is not behaviorally controlled to minimize discomfort. In all of our studies, we failed to disprove the hypothesis that air hunger is caused by a parallel copy of increased brainstem respiratory motor activity ('corollary discharge'). Finally, hypercapnia induced air hunger modified but never fully suppressed the ability to behaviorally control breathing for purposes of speech.

ACKNOWLEDGMENTS

Most of the work referred to in this review chapter has been performed in close collaboration with Robert B Banzett PhD, Physiology Program, Harvard School of Public Health, Boston, M A 02115, USA, and funded by US. Public Health Service Grants from the Heart, Lung and Blood Institute, principally Grant # HL 46690. Other collaborators have included Andy Andres, Elisabeth Bloch-Salisbury PhD, Robert Brown MD, Karleyton Evans, Abraham Guz MD, Helen Harty, PhD, Jeanette D. Hoit PhD, Harold Manning MD, Daniel Shannon MD, Christina M Spengler PhD, and David Systrom MD.

REFERENCES

1. Shea SA, Lansing RW, Banzett RB (1995) Respiratory sensations and their role in the control of breathing. In: Regulation of Breathing, Dempsey JA, Pack AI (eds.) In the series: Lung Biology in Health and Disease, Lenfant, C (ed.). Marcel Dekker, New York, pp.xx-xx

2. Banzett RB, Lansing RW, Evans KC, Shea SA (1996) Stimulus-response characteristics of CO2 induced air hunger in normal subjects. Respir. Physiol. 103:19-31

3. Shea SA, Evans KC (1994) Time course of changes in air hunger following altered ventilator tidal volume. FASEB J. 8:A271.

4. Manning H, Shea SA, Schwartzstein R, Lansing RW, Brown R, Banzett RB (1992) Decreased tidal volume increases `air hunger' at constant PCO2 in ventilated C1-C3 quadriplegics. Respir Physiol. 90:19-30

5. Bloch-Salisbury E, Shea SA, Brown R, Evans, K, Banzett RB (1996) Air hunger induced by acute hypercapnia adapts to chronic hypercapnia in ventilated humans. J. Appl. Physiol. 81:949-956

6. Shea SA. Relationship between subject-selected tidal volume and air hunger sensation during hypercapnia in humans (1996) Am. J. Respir. & Crit. Care Med. 153: A116

7. Shea SA, Harty HR, Banzett RB (1996) Self-control of level of mechanical ventilation to minimize CO2-induced air hunger. Respir. Physiol. 103:113-125

8. Shea SA, Andres LP, Shannon DC, Guz A, Banzett RB (1993) Respiratory sensations in subjects who lack a ventilatory response to CO2. Respir Physiol. 93:203-219

9. Spengler CM, Banzett RB, Systrom DM, Shannon DC, Shea SA (1998) Respiratory sensations during heavy exercise in subjects without ventilatory chemosensitivity. Respir. Physiol. 114: 65-74

10. Shea SA, Hoit JD, Banzett RB (1998) Competition between gas exchange and speech production in ventilated subjects. Biol. Psychol. 49: 9-27

Dyspnea in patients with asthma

Yoshihiro Kikuchi, Shinichi Okabe, Hajime Kurosawa, Hiromasa Ogawa, Wataru Hida, and Kunio Shirato

The First Department of Internal Medicine, Tohoku University School of Medicine, 1-1 Seiryo-machi Aoba-ku, Sendai 980-8574, Japan

Summary: Dyspnea may be one of the defense systems of our body, like pain or other sensations. Accordingly, if the perception of dyspnea is lost or blunted in patients with asthma, it could be dangerous. In this study, to examine the mechanisms of death from asthma and to elucidate the important role of the dyspnea sensation in preventing death from asthmatic attack, we performed two studies. First, we examined the perception of dyspnea and the chemosensitivity to hypoxia and hypercapnia in 11 patients with a history of near-fatal asthma (NFA). Second, we also examined circumstances of life-threatening attacks or triggering factors of unconsciousness by interviewing 20 patients with NFA. The hypoxic responses of patients with NFA were significantly decreased as compared with those of the normal subjects and the patients with usual asthma. By contrast, there were no significant differences in the hypercapnic responses among the three groups. Dyspnea sensation measured with the Borg score while breathing though graded resistances, was also significantly lower in the patients with NFA than in the normal subjects. In addition, most of the patients with NFA had lost consciousness due to increasing physical activity or inhalation of β_2-stimulants through an ultrasonic nebulizer. They did not feel severe suffocation before losing consciousness. These results suggest that (1) lowered hypoxic chemosensitivity and blunted perception of dyspnea may predispose patients to life-threatening attacks and that (2) severe hypoxemia induced by increasing physical activity may be a primary cause of losing consciousness, leading to death.

Key word. Death from asthma, Near-fatal asthma, Hypoxic ventilatory response, Blunted perception of dyspnea, Defence mechanisms

INTRODUCTION

Bronchial asthma is characterized by an increased responsiveness of the airway to various stimuli and by various degrees of widespread narrowing of the airway. The narrowing of the airway is usually reversible, and during an exacerbation, the patient suffers from various degrees of an uncomfortable sensation in breathing or dyspnea due to bronchoconstriction. Thus, dyspnea is usually an unpleasant sensation for the patients with asthma. On the other hand, however, the sensation of dyspnea is regarded as one of the defense systems of our body, such as pain or other sensations. Dyspnea would give warning to the patients when their respiratory condition is abnormal or dangerous. Therefore, if the patient's perception of dyspnea is blunted or lost, it might be potentially dangerous because the severity of an exacerbation of asthma may be underestimated [1-4]. However, this possibility has not been thoroughly examined, although it has been repeatedly demonstrated that the perception of airway narrowing is blunted in some asthmatic patients [3]. The purpose of the present study was to examine the mechanism of death from asthma, and to show the important relationship between the perceptibility of the dyspnea sensation and death from asthmatic attack.

What is the mechanism of death from asthma or of fatal asthmatic attack? Although there are many studies regarding this issue [5-7] , the mechanism of fatal attack has not been fully determined yet. Molfino et al. [8] have reported that respiratory arrest, not cardiac arrest, may be the principal cause of death during attack. However, the underlying causes of respiratory arrest have not been elucidated yet. As risk factors of death, several matters such as low compliance for medication, smoking, aging etc. have been reported [9]. However, most of these seem non-specific, and the most reliable risk factor seems to be a previous history of near-fatal attack [1].

To clarify the mechanisms of fatal attacks, we performed two studies. In the first study, we measured the perception of dyspnea and the chemosensitivity to hypoxia and hypercapnia in patients with a history of near-fatal asthma. Several epidemiological studies have shown that patients with near-fatal asthma have characteristics similar to those of the patients who died of asthma and that they are at high risk for a subsequent and possibly fatal attack [6- 7]. It follows that studies of near-fatal asthma may provide insight for clarifying the mechanisms of death from asthma. Our hypothesis was that the dyspnea sensation and/or chemosensitivity may be blunted in some patients with asthma. Therefore, their responses to airway obstruction may not be sufficient to protect them from profound hypoxia and hypercapnia.

In the second study, to elucidate the direct triggering factors for unconsciousness, we examined the circumstances of life-threatening attacks or triggering factors of unconsciousness by interviewing twenty patients with near fatal asthma.

The greater part of the study has been already reported in the journal [10].

STUDY 1: CHEMOSENSITIVITY AND DYSPNEA IN PATIENTS WITH NEAR-FATAL ASTHMA.

Methods of Study 1:
Subjects: The subjects were 11 patients who had near-fatal asthma attacks (NFA) (mean age 39), 11 patients with asthma who had no experience of near-fatal attacks (usual asthma) (mean age 32), and 16 normals (mean age 33). Patients more than 62 yr or less than 18 yr were excluded from this experiment. Patients with NFA were defined as those with asthma who had become unconsciousness with severe respiratory failure during an attack of asthma (three patients) or had undergone mechanical ventilation during an asthma exacerbation (eight subjects). Patients with usual asthma were defined as those who had had no near-fatal attacks. The arterial blood gas values indicated that severe respiratory failure with retention of carbon dioxide had occurred during their latest near-fatal attacks. Five of the 11 patients had had more than one near-fatal attack.

To exclude the possible effect of airway obstruction on the measurements of chemosensitivity and the sensation of dyspnea, the patients were enrolled in this study when their disease was clinically diagnosed as in remission as evidenced by no rales, wheezing nor dyspnea attacks for at least three weeks before the study, and when the forced expiratory volume in one second (FEV$_1$) was greater than 80 percent of the predicted value. The sensation of dyspnea during resistive loading was not measured in four normal subjects who were familiar with the purpose of this study. The investigation was approved by the Institutional Ethics Committee, and informed consent was obtained from all the subjects.

Protocols and Measurements: After spirometry and plethysmographic measurements of airway resistance, the perceptibility of dyspnea during inspiratory resistive loading and chemosensitivity to hypoxia and hypercapnia were measured using a previously described apparatus consisting of a unidirectional Hans-Rudolph valve and a rebreathing circuit [11]. Mouth pressure was measured with a Validyne pressure transducer, which was used with a device to obtain airway occlusion pressures (P$_{0.1}$, the mouth pressure 0.1 second after onset of inspiration against an occluded airway)[12]. Minute ventilation (V$_E$) was measured by electrically integrating the expiratory flow signal. End-tidal carbon dioxide tension (P$_{ET}$CO$_2$) and end-tidal oxygen tension (P$_{ET}$O$_2$) were monitored with a mass spectrometer. Arterial oxygen saturation (SaO$_2$) was measured continuously with a finger pulse oximeter.

The sensation of dyspnea was measured while the subject breathed through linear inspiratory resistances of 0 (control), 2.3, 5.0, 10.1, 20.0, and 30.9 centimeters of water per liter per second. Neither ventilation nor breathing pattern was controlled during the test. After one-minute breathing through each resistance, the subject rated the intensity of the sensation of discomfort of breathing (dyspnea) by using a modified Borg scale [13]. This is a category scale in which the subject selects a number describing the magnitude of the sensation of dyspnea ranging from 0 (no difficulty breathing) to 10 (maximal difficulty breathing). The term discomfort of breathing was not defined any further, but the subjects were instructed to avoid rating non-respiratory sensations such as headache or irritation of the pharynx.

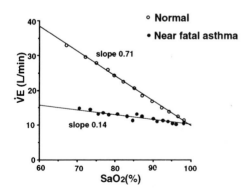

Fig. 1. Representative Responses to Hypoxia in One Normal Subject and One Patient with Near-Fatal Asthma. These two responses were chosen because their slope values were the median of each group. The normal subject increased ventilation with the decrease in arterial oxygen saturation. The slope of the normal subject was 0.71. By contrast, the patient with near-fatal asthma increased ventilation only slightly and the slope was 0.14. This value is about one-fifth of the normal subject's value.

Respiratory responses to progressive isocapnic hypoxia and progressive hyperoxic hypercapnia were measured using standard rebreathing methods [14, 15], and were assessed in terms of slopes of ventilation and airway occlusion pressure as a function of P$_{ET}$CO2 and SaO2. After an equilibration period while breathing room air, the subjects rebreathed through a bag containing the initial gas mixture: 21 percent oxygen in nitrogen for the hypoxic response and 7 percent carbon dioxide in oxygen for the hypercapnic response. In the hypoxic test, a

34

bypass circuit consisting of a carbon dioxide-absorber and a variable fan was connected between the inspiratory and expiratory lines, and $P_{ET}CO_2$ was held constant (within ± 1 mmHg) at the level of each subject's resting $P_{ET}CO2$ during the procedure by varying the flow of the carbon dioxide-absorber. The trials of hypoxic and hypercapnic responses were terminated when the subjects reached 70 percent SaO_2 and 64 mmHg $P_{ET}CO2$, respectively.

Results are expressed as Mean$\pm$SD. The slopes of the ventilatory and airway occlusion pressure responses to hypercapnia and hypoxia were calculated by the method of least-squares regression analysis to $P_{ET}CO_2$ and SaO_2, respectively. Statistical analysis for comparisons was done using a one-way analysis of variance and a two-tailed Student's t-test, and a two-way analysis of variance with a post hoc Scheffe's test. P values of less than 0.05 were considered significant.

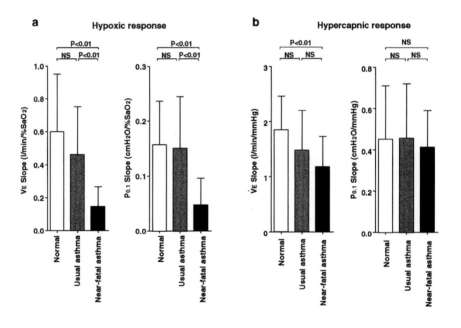

Fig. 2. a. Mean Values ($\pm$SD) of Hypoxic Response Expressed in Terms of Ventilatory (V_E) Slope ($\Delta V_E/\Delta SaO_2$)(left) and Airway Occlusion Pressure ($P_{0.1}$) Slope ($\Delta P_{0.1}/\Delta SaO_2$)(right) in Normals, Patients with Usual Asthma, and Patients with Near-Fatal Asthma. Note that patients with near-fatal asthma had low slope values for both V_E and $P_{0.1}$. Both the mean values of the ventilatory and $P_{0.1}$ slopes were significantly lower in the patients with near-fatal asthma than in the normal subjects (P<0.01 for both slopes) and also than patients with usual asthma (P<0.01 for both slopes).
b. Mean Values ($\pm$SD) of Hyperoxic Hypercapnic Responses Expressed in Terms of Ventilatory (V_E) Slope ($\Delta V_E/\Delta P_{ET}CO_2$)(left) and Airway Occlusion Pressure ($P_{0.1}$) Slope ($\Delta P_{0.1}/\Delta P_{ET}CO_2$)(right) in the Three Groups. The mean value of $\Delta V_E/\Delta P_{ET}CO_2$ in the patients with near-fatal asthma was significantly different from that of the normal subjects (P<0.01), but not from that of patients with usual asthma. By contrast, there were no significant differences in the mean values of $\Delta P_{0.1}/\Delta P_{ET}CO_2$ among these three groups.

Results of Study 1:
There was no significant difference in the mean duration of asthma between the two asthma groups, and similar drugs were used for the treatment of asthma in the two asthma groups. Spirometry was within the normal range in the all patients.   There were no significant differences in the Raw values between the two asthmatic groups.

Figure 1 shows representative responses to hypoxia in one normal subject and one patient with near-fatal asthma. These two responses were chosen because their slope values were the median of each group. In the normal subject, ventilation increased with the decrease in arterial oxygen saturation. The value of his slope was 0.71. By contrast, in this patient with near-fatal asthma, ventilation increased only slightly and the value of the slope was 0.14. This value is about one-fifth of the normal subject's value.

Figure 2a shows the mean values of the hypoxic responses in normals, patients with usual asthma, and patients with near-fatal asthma. Both the mean values of the ventilatory and $P_{0.1}$ slopes were significantly lower in the patients with near-fatal asthma than those in normals and also than patients with usual asthma. Figure 2b shows the mean values of hypercapnic responses expressed in terms of the ventilatory slope on the left and the $P_{0.1}$ slope on the right. The mean value of the ventilatory slope in patients with near-fatal asthma was significantly different from that of normals, but not from that of patients with usual asthma. By contrast, there were no significant differences in the mean values of the $P_{0.1}$ slope among these three groups.

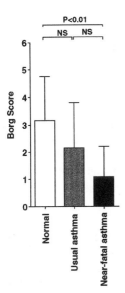

Fig. 3. The Mean Values (±SD) of the Borg Score During Breathing with a Resistance of 20.0 $cmH_2O/l/sec$ in the three groups. The mean values in the patients with near-fatal asthma were significantly different from those in the normal subjects (Scheffe's test; $P<0.01$), but not different from those in the patients with usual asthma. There was no significant difference between the mean values of the patients with usual asthma and the normal subjects.

The mean values of the Borg score obtained during breathing through a resistance of 20 $cmH_2O/liter/sec$ are shown in Fig. 3. In patients with usual asthma, there was a non-significant decrease from the mean values of the Borg score from normals. The mean value of the Borg score in patients with near-fatal asthma was significantly lower than that of normals.

STUDY 2: TRIGGERING FACTORS FOR UNCONSCIOUSNESS.

Methods of Study 2:
The subjects were 20 patients with NFA (mean age 38). They had had an experience of near-fatal asthma attack in the past 7 years. All 20 patients had recovered well from their life-threatening attacks. Their disease was controlled well thereafter using their regular treatment. Eight of the patients had been measured the chemosensitivity and dyspnea in the "Study 1".

All patients were interviewed directly by us when they visited or while they were in the hospital. Specifically, we asked the following:
(1) the precise situation or subject's behavior before losing consciousness,
(2) whether they used β_2-stimulant inhalation before losing consciousness,
(3) whether they felt severe suffocation, possibly severe enough to threaten their lives.

Result of Study 2:
All patients could remember well about their situation and circumstances when they had lost consciousness. Fourteen patients lost consciousness relatively suddenly (within several minutes), during or just after increasing physical activity, in most cases, walking. Three patients lost consciousness during inhalation of β_2-stimulants through an electrically driven ultrasonic nebulizer. The other three patients were in an ambulance or a relative's car.

Fourteen patients, although they noticed their attacks and felt some dyspneic sensation, denied having a feeling of severe suffocation. Thirteen of these fourteen were the patients who lost consciousness while engaging in or just after increasing physical activity.

DISCUSSION

The results of our study demonstrate that most of the patients with NFA have lowered hypoxic chemosensitivity as well as a blunted sensation of dyspnea during resistive loading compared with normal subjects and patients with usual asthma. In addition, most of the patients with NFA had lost consciousness due to increasing physical activity or inhalation of β_2-stimulants through an ultrasonic nebulizer. They did not feel severe suffocation before losing consciousness.

The important underlying assumption that we used in this study was that the pathophysiologic processes in patients who did die from asthma attack are similar to those occurring in our patients with near-fatal asthma attacks. Obviously, this assumption is not necessarily correct and one may claim that we were observing a so-called survivor effect. However, epidemiological reports [6, 7] repeatedly emphasized that many patients who die of asthma had preceding near-fatal asthmatic attacks, which tends to support our assumption that our patients with near-fatal asthma are probably representative of a subgroup of patients with fatal asthma.

Since Rubinfield and Pain's [3] important observation that perception of airway narrowing is blunted in some asthmatics, there have been relatively few studies which investigated this further. Although it is speculated that such a decreased perception may be potentially dangerous because the severity of an exacerbation may be underestimated [1, 2, 4], this possibility had never been systematically examined. We have found that, although there was a wide variation of the individual values of the Borg score among all subjects, most patients with near-fatal asthma have a markedly depressed perception of dyspnea during inspiratory resistive loading. These results suggest that, when such patients feel dyspnea, the degree of their airway obstruction might already be very severe.

Our findings that most patients had a lowered hypoxic response accompanied by a blunted sensation of dyspnea and/or lowered hypercapnic response suggest that, in addition to severe bronchoconstriction due to an exacerbation of asthma, a lack of or decreased defense mechanisms against profound hypoxia, hypercapnia and airway narrowing may play an important role in causing life-threatening asthma attacks. Although MacFadden [1] and Hudgel [2] stated that, if chemosensitivity is blunted in asthmatics, the patients may possibly develop severe respiratory failure leading to death, this speculation had not been systematically examined yet.

Several reports suggest that the ability to respond to hypoxia might be influenced by a hereditary factor, presumably a genetic one [16-19]. Weil and Hudgel [16] have demonstrated that some family members of their asthmatic patients who have a lowered hypoxic response and repeated severe respiratory failure during asthma exacerbations, also have a lowered hypoxic response, suggesting that the diminished hypoxic response might be determined genetically. Thus it seems possible that the lowered hypoxic response observed in our patients with NFA may be inherited genetically rather than secondarily acquired as a result of repeated hypoxic exposure. It is well established that the most important factor in the control of ventilation is CO_2 tension in the arterial blood and that the role of the hypoxic stimulus in the usual control of ventilation is small [20]. Thus, it is not surprising that the patients with NFA are usually quite normal during off-attack periods, even if they do not increase ventilation during hypoxic exposure. However, it is assumed that, in the unusual condition where hypoxemia is progressing, for example at high altitude [21], the ability to respond to hypoxia may play a critical role in maintaining breathing. We thus speculate that this may be the case in life-threatening asthma attacks. A very similar situation has been proposed as one of the mechanisms involved in sudden infant death syndrome [22].

To elucidate further the mechanisms of death from asthma, we interviewed the patients with NFA and asked about the precise situation when they had lost consciousness. Seventy percent of our patients with NFA had lost consciousness during or just after increasing physical activity and 15% had lost it after or during inhalation of β_2-stimulants through an ultrasonic nebulizer. It is likely that such exercise, even if very mild, might make their hypoxemia more serious during severe attacks. It is also established that inhalation of β_2-stimulants during attacks decreases arterial oxygen tension (20). In addition, our findings that most patients relatively suddenly (within minutes) lost consciousness indicate that severe hypoxemia might be the primary cause of unconsciousness rather than hypercapnia, which usually induces the loss of consciousness more gradually. Moreover, although they of course noticed their attacks and were feeling some dyspneic sensation, these patients denied having a feeling of severe suffocation. These results strongly suggest that unconsciousness was induced by severe hypoxemia rather than asphyxiation during the life-threatening asthma attacks. If the main cause for losing consciousness is profound hypoxemia which is induced by increasing physical activity, both the lowered hypoxic response and the blunted perception of dyspnea would be responsible for suvh life-threatening attacks of asthma. This may be the reason why most of our patients with NFA showed both of them.

In summary, we have examined the mechanisms by which fatal or near-fatal asthma attacks develop in patients with NFA. Most of these subjects had a lowered hypoxic response as well as a lowered sensation of dyspnea during resistive loading. Moreover, they had lost consciousness during or after increasing physical activity without a feeling of severe dyspnea. These results suggest that severe hypoxemia rather than asphyxiation may be the primary cause for the unconsciousness during a life-threatening asthmatic attack.

REFERENCES

1. McFadden ER Jr. (1991) Fatal and near-fatal asthma. N Engl J Med 324:409-10.
2. Hudgel DW (1985) Control of breathing in asthma. In: Weiss EB, Segal MS, Stein M, eds. Bronchial Asthma 2nd ed. Little, Brown, Boston, pp193-8.
3. Rubinfield AR, Pain CF (1976) Perception of asthma. Lancet 1:882-884.
4. Barnes PJ (1992) Poorly perceived asthma. Thorax 47:408-9.
5. British Thoracic Association (1982) Death from asthma in two regions of England. Br Med J 285:1251-5.
6. Sears MR, Rea HH (1987) Patients at risk for dying of asthma: New Zealand Experience. J Allergy Clin Immunol 80:477-81.
7. Rea HH, Scragg R, Jackson R, Beaglehole R, Fenwick J, Sutherland D (1986) A case-control study of death from asthma. Thorax 41:833-9.
8. Molfino NA, Nannini LJ, Martelli AN, Slutsky AS (1991) Respiratory arrest in near-fatal asthma. N Engl J Med 324:285-8.
9. Benatar SR (1986) Fatal asthma. N Engl J Med 314:423-9.
10. Kikuchi Y, Okabe S, Tamura G, Hida W, Homma M, Shirato K, Takishima T (1994) Chemosensitivity and perception of dyspnea in patients with a history of near-fatal asthma. N Engl J Med 330: 1329-34.
11. Taguchi O, Kikuchi Y, Hida W, et al (1991) Effects of bronchoconstriction and external resistive loading on the sensation of dyspnea. J Appl Physiol 71:2183-90.
12 .Whitelaw W, Derenne JP, Milic-Emili J (1975) Occlusion pressure as a measure of respiratory center output in conscious man. Respir Physiol 23: 181-99.
13. El-Manshawi A, Killian KJ, Summers E, Jones NJ (1986) Breathlessness during exercise with and without resistive loading. J Appl Physiol 61: 895-905.
14. Read DJC (1967) A clinical method for assessing the ventilatory response to CO_2. Aust Ann Med 16:22-32.
15. Rebuck AS, Campbell EJM. (1974) A clinical method for assessing the ventilatory response to hypoxia. Am Rev Respir Dis 109:345-50.
16. Hudgel DW, Weil JV (1974) Asthma associated with decreased hypoxic ventilatory drive: a family study. Ann Intern Med 80:623-5.
17. Collins DD, Scoggin CH, Zwillich CW, Weil JV (1978) Hereditary aspect of decreased hypoxic response. J Clin Invest 62:105-10.
18. Moore GC, Zwillich CW, Battaglia JD, Cotton EK, Weil JV (1976) Respiratory failure associated with familial depression of ventilatory response to hypoxia and hypercapnia. N Engl J Med 295:861-5.

19. Kawakami Y, Yoshikawa T, Shida A, Asamuma Y, Murao M (1982) Control of breathing in young twins. J Appl Physiol 52:537-42.
20. West JB (1985) Respiratory Physiology, the essentials. 3rd Eds. Williams and Wilkins , Baltimore, pp113-27.
21. Lakshminarayan S, Pierson DJ (1975) Recurrent high altitude pulmonary edema with blunted chemosensitivity. Am Rev Respir Dis 111:869-72.
22. Hunt CE, McCulloch K, Broullette RT (1981) Diminished hypoxic ventilatory responses in near-miss sudden infant death syndrome. J Appl Physiol 50:1313-7.

Respiration and Emotion (I)

How Breathing Adjusts to Mental and Physical Demands

Paul Grossman[1] and Cees J. Wientjes[2]

[1]Breathing Space: Institute for Yoga, Meditation and Health, Konradstrasse 32, 79100 Freiburg, Germany, and HRCA Laboratory for Cardiovascular Research, Boston, MA, USA
[2]TNO Human Factors Research Institute, Soesterburg, the Netherlands

Summary

Psychological influences upon respiratory regulation remain a much neglected area of investigation, although it is apparent that parameters of breathing must be integrated into a wide range of behavioral, emotional and cognitive acts. The general lack of knowledge regarding respiratory adjustments to psychological demands has led to the assumption that limited and stereotyped changes in respiratory variables are characteristic across the range of mental/emotional activities. However, this belief is not consistent with the rich and highly variable respiratory responses that can be demonstrated in the laboratory. Our research has examined the effects upon breathing of a wide variety of cognitive/emotional and physical demands, employing non-intrusive assessment of timing and volumetric components of the respiratory pattern. The findings indicate that dynamic and specific changes of breathing are uniquely related to the task-specific properties, whether primarily psychological or physical in nature. Given (1) the important function of breathing in mediating rapid, continuous changes in metabolic demands, (2) the integrated mid- and higher-brain control of breathing, and (3) our awareness and conscious sensitivity to ventilatory parameters, we believe that respiratory adjustments to highly specific behavioral demands have evolved as functional integrative adaptations to best fit and coordinate metabolic activity, cognitive performance, emotional self-regulation and perhaps even communicative signaling to conspecifics. Nevertheless, why the breathing pattern changes as it does to certain psychological circumstances remains highly speculative and unclear. Plausible hypotheses remain uncharted territory, and future investigation should focus upon the specific cognitive, emotional, signaling and metabolic demands of varying psychological demands, as well as brain centers controlling breathing under these variable conditions.

Introduction

The investigation of respiration in relation to psychological phenomena remains one of the truly neglected areas of psychophysiology, behavioral medicine and neurophysiology. Respiration, of all major physiological processes, would appear to be, perhaps, the most obvious candidate to examine in association with psychological demands. Specific respiratory symptoms are frequently reported to emotionally stressful states, a sudden scare takes the breath out of each of us, we can easily observe the connection in ourselves or among others between certain states of consciousness and changes in breathing (e.g. sleep-wake differences or acute fear), and we know that the particulars of speaking and other behavioral activities must be coordinated with our breathing. Furthermore, it has been evident for over half a century that ventilation is under the control of higher, mid-brain and lower centers of the central nervous system, and somehow central integration of voluntary and automatic aspects of ventilation must be organized in a sophisticated but as yet unclear manner. Most recently, aspects of respiratory control have been implicated in the development or maintenance of major clinical anxiety disorders [1,2]. Nevertheless, breathing parameters remain, at best, control variables in psychophysiological investigations, probably due to just the fact that respiration is so available to awareness. Possibly, also the lack of obvious disease states associated with the interface between psychology and variations in respiratory pattern may have impeded sufficient funding (with the exception of bronchial asthma focusing on abnormal airway resistance). Whatever the causes, this situation has led to a extremely sluggish pace in the advancement of respiratory psychophysiology over the last several decades [3].

Our own respiratory research has examined psychophysiological aspects of ventilatory pattern in both health and disease [4-6] focusing upon parameters of timing, volume and metabolic appropriateness of breathing during performance of stressful mental tasks. Our earlier investigations primarily indicated that patients with hyperventilation syndrome, in contrast to matched controls, showed no abnormalities in respiratory pattern nor hyperventilation during psychological stress but did report many more somatic symptoms often considered suggestive of hyperventilation (summarized in [4]). On the other hand, we have consistently found that reduced levels of end-tidal carbon dioxide in the laboratory are associated with chronic anxiety and enhanced report of psychosomatic symptoms [7]. In this chapter, however, we will review our normative findings relating ventilatory parameters to specific psychological task demands in the laboratory. Unlike most psychophysiological investigators of breathing, we have not only compared qualitatively different cognitive/emotional tasks but have also examined variations in breathing pattern when subtle, quantitatively explicit task parameters are manipulated (e.g. accuracy and speed of performance). Thus, we have been able to see whether a gradient of respiratory response occurs as particular psychological demands increase in magnitude, as well as how the basic biological respiratory function of meeting ever-changing metabolic demand is simultaneously coordinated.

Our studies typically include a relatively fine-grained analysis of both timing and volumetric aspects of breathing shown in Figure 1, derived from non-intrusive measurement employing two calibrated inductive plethysmographic chest bands (Respitrace). In addition, end-tidal carbon dioxide via capnograph—an index of eucapnia, hyperventilation and hypocapnia—and the ratio of abdominal-to-thoracic contribution to tidal volume is often assessed. In order to maintain brevity, we will mainly explore the timing and volumetric parameters in this presentation.

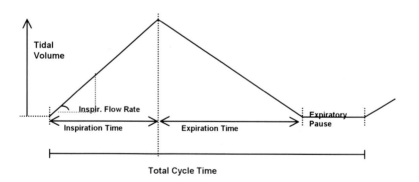

Figure 1. Time and Volume Components of the Breathing Cycle

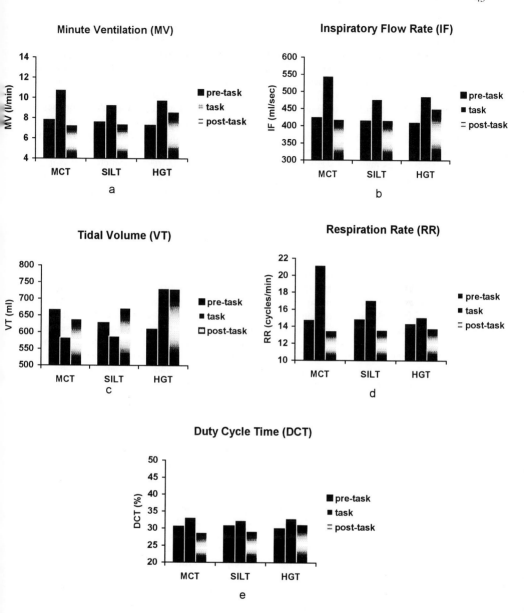

Figure 2. Respiratory parameters in Study 1: Mean levels in response to the memory comparison task (MCT), the silhouette task (SILT) and isometric handgrip (HGT).

We will now review a series of four studies with varying psychological and physical task demands using healthy adult subjects. Our major objectives are to describe the manner by which ventilation accommodates metabolic, behavioral and cognitive-emotional demands under a wide range of real-life conditions: How are metabolically necessary changes in minute and alveolar ventilation achieved under differing circumstances? Alterations in minute ventilation (liters of air inspired per minute) can be accomplished by various means, i.e. changes in respiration rate, tidal volume, duty cycle (ratio of inspiration time to expiration time) and/or inspiratory flow (the rate of air inspired per second); are there similar minute ventilatory responses to different tasks, and are these achieved by similar or different adjustments of these other parameters? In other words, are there distinctive breathing patterns for differing emotional/cognitive states that mediate metabolic requirements? We hope that our findings may be a starting point in explicating (1) why respiration changes as it does in response to specific emotional and/or cognitive demands, and (2) whether chronic disturbances of emotion (e.g. anxiety disorders) are meaningfully related to specific respiratory alterations in a causal manner.

Study 1: Repetitive Mental Tasks and Isometric Exercise

In this study, we investigated 50 adult male subjects (30-40 years old) during performance of two quite different and challenging five-minute reaction-time tasks, both requiring very rapid positive or negative responses with the same stimulus-response characteristics (e.g. maximal duration of stimulus presentation 1500 ms, and succeeding trials 200 ms after previous response or default no-response (i.e. 1000 ms without response): (1) a five minute memory-comparison task (MCT) in which subjects were required to compare a visual display of four letters for presence or absence of a previously memorized set of two letters; (2) A silhouette task (SILT) in which ambiguous geometric shapes were compared for magnitude of area without real possibility for accurate determination, and apparent negative feedback (100-Hz white noise) was presented randomly averaging every tenth trial. Additionally, ventilatory patterns of activity were examined during a period of isometric handgrip (HGT) at 75% maximal force. Each condition was preceded by pre- and post-task baselines (task conditions, counterbalanced order). The results are presented in Figure 2a-e.

Minute ventilation increased from baseline levels for each task condition. There were no significant differences in degree of minute ventilation response among the three conditions, although mean elevation was highest for the MCT; employing a 160-ml correction for dead-space ventilation and adjusting alveolar ventilation for respiration rate, MCT and HGT task levels were almost identical, and both about 1.5 liters higher than for the SILT task. End-tidal CO_2 partial pressure ($P_{et}CO_2$; not shown) was not altered from baseline, indicating that the minute ventilation volume changes reflected real increases in task-related metabolic activity, and the extent of metabolic change was the same for all tasks, with SILT inducing modestly less metabolic activity. On the other hand, quite different patterns of respiratory activity were employed to achieve largely the same enhancement of ventilation appropriate to metabolic activity. Thus, respiration rate increased from baseline to each both mental tasks, although less pronounced for SILT; respiration rate was not altered during HGT. Tidal volume, in contrast, showed similar reductions from baseline for both reaction-time tasks, but actually increased relatively dramatically during handgrip. Inspiratory flow rate, an index of central respiratory drive, increased for all tasks, but the sole difference between task conditions was a greater elevation during MCT. Duty cycle, an index of central timing of ventilation, manifested a similarly very slight but significant increase from baseline to each task phase.

These results, therefore, indicate that different patterns of breathing subserve similar changes in ventilation required to meet alterations in metabolic demand during isometric physical exercise and moderate mental activity. During repetitive cognitive performance, minute ventilation increase was achieved primarily by a rise in respiration rate, a decrease in tidal volume and enhancement of inspiratory flow rate (especially so for the MCT where ventilation and presumably metabolic

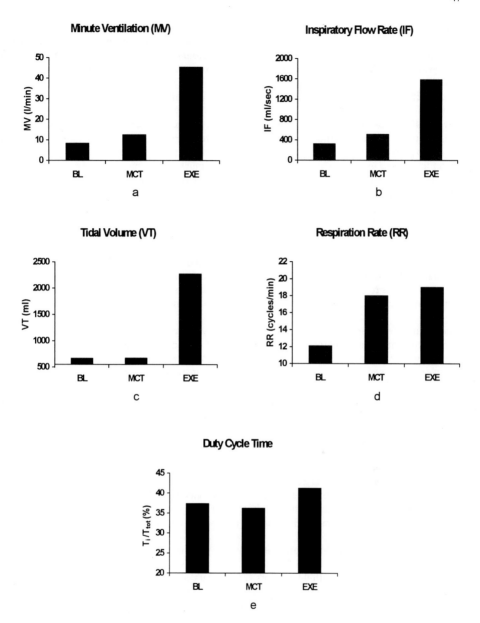

Figure 3. Respiratory parameters in Study 2: Mean levels during baseline (BL), memory-comparison task (MCT), and 100-Watt ergometer exercise (EXE).

activity was most elevated). Isometric exercise, however, was characterized by a similar increase of minute and alveolar ventilation, mediated by a sizeable *increase* of tidal volume, moderate rise in inspiratory flow rate and no change in respiration rate from resting baseline. The next investigation will explore how moderate *aerobic* activity compares to repetitive mental performance.

Study 2: Repetitive Mental Performance Vs. Aerobic Activity

Twenty 40-50 year-old adults performed a five-minute period of the previously described MCT and a 5-min phase of bicycle ergometry at 100-watts exercise intensity [8]. Figures 2a-e illustrate the major findings (BL, baseline). Note that both tasks increase minute ventilation, with a much larger effect for aerobic exercise. This, of course, reflects the much greater metabolic demand of 100-watt exercise compared to mental activity. Once again, dynamic exercise, like isometric handgrip, increased minute ventilation primarily by means of much enhanced tidal volume, accompanied by a moderate increase in respiration rate. Respiration rate, in fact, was very similar between tasks, and there was no significant difference between the two task conditions. Inspiratory flow rate increased from baseline for both tasks, although this parameter was far greater during dynamic exercise than MCT. As in Study 1, absence of effects upon $P_{et}CO_2$ indicated that minute ventilation increases during tasks were proportional to elevations in metabolic activity. The lack of difference in respiration rate, furthermore, pointed to alterations in tidal volume, alone, accounting for ventilatory accommodations to metabolic requirements during both tasks. In contrast to all other conditions of both reported studies, duty cycle increased substantially during dynamic exercise.

The findings from these first two investigations clearly demonstrate that both mental and physical demands elevate minute ventilation to meet metabolic demands, although it is clear that repetitive mental activity elicits much more modest metabolic increases than even mild-to-moderate dynamic exercise. With isometric exercise, the relatively small increases in oxygen demand are mediated solely by tidal-volume contribution to minute ventilation. With dynamic exercise, a more pronounced rise in metabolic activity is accommodated by a larger elevation of tidal volume and an increase in respiration rate, the latter being similar to that during mental performance. During mental tasks, the small elevations of metabolic activity were completely mediated by the contribution of increased respiration rate to minute ventilation; tidal volume actually decreased during mental stress, although only slightly in Study 2. These results could indicate that either (1) there is a fundamental difference in ventilatory regulation between repetitive tasks requiring primarily physical *vs.* mental engagement, or (2) ventilatory patterns are primarily sensitive to the level of metabolic demand, the greater the oxygen demand the more tidal volume is recruited. The next investigation attempted simultaneously to alter both mental load and metabolic activity in order to examine effects upon breathing pattern and minute ventilation.

Study 3: Motivational Manipulation of the Memory-Comparison Task

This study was performed with 44 students (21-30 years old), employing the previously described MCT using substantial monetary reward as motivation for good performance [6]. Three different conditions were presented to all subjects: (1) a no-feedback condition (NFB) in which no information was presented to subjects regarding accuracy or speed of performance (20 min); (2) a feedback condition (FB) in which visual information was presented after each trial regarding whether subjects met criteria of speed and accuracy (20 min; conditions 1 and 2 counterbalanced for order); and (3) a so-called "all-or-nothing" condition (AON; 10 min), always presented last, in which subjects were required--in order for them to keep their previous winnings--to perform better than during any of the prior conditions. Performance standards were first set during a training phase prior to the actual experiment, then automatically computer updated every five minutes. The algorithm employed a combined criteria of speed and accuracy. Subjects were able to make as much as $25 with good performance.

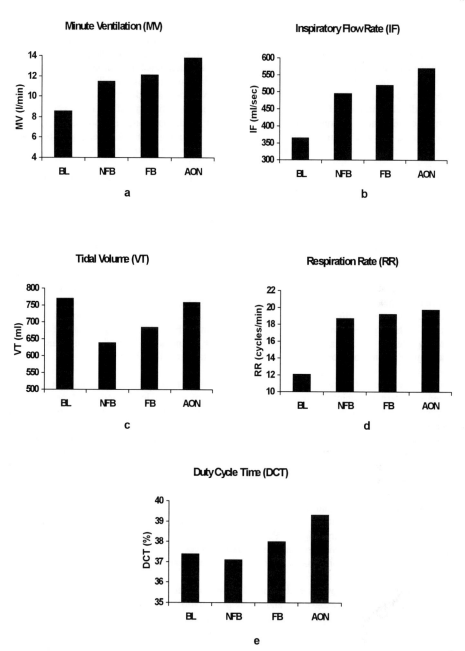

Figure 4. Respiratory parameters in Study 3: Mean levels during baseline (BL), no-feedback (NFB), feedback (FB)and all-or-nothing (AON) conditions of the memory comparison task

Because the task remained the same during all conditions, we assumed that differences in performance would be a consequence of variations in motivational state, although we could not exclude other factors (e.g. differences in stressfulness or elicitation of distinct emotional states between conditions). Nevertheless, we believed that a gradient of performance improvement corresponding to task condition would best be explained by motivational state. These manipulations were performed with the hypothesis that feedback of information would provide greater motivation than no feedback, and the AON condition would be the most motivating of all. However, no clear performance differences emerged between NFB and FB conditions, since an increase in speed of reaction during FB was counteracted by a decrease in accuracy. On the other hand, the AON condition showed large performance improvement compared with both other tasks.

Examination of the respiratory data (Figures 3a-e) indicates a significant monotonic increase of minute ventilation from baseline through the AON condition (all condition differences significant). Absence of respiration rate and $P_{et}CO_2$ differences between task conditions indicates that alveolar ventilation and metabolic demand increased linearly across performance conditions, as well, of course, as showing changes from baseline. Hence, we were able to significantly manipulate metabolic activity within a single repetitive mental load paradigm by altering performance, most likely via motivational change. Breathing pattern was also altered across task conditions in a characteristic manner: Respiration rate increased from baseline to all performance conditions, but did not differ among the MCT conditions. In contrast, tidal volume decreased from baseline to NFB, rose during FB and actually achieved a level comparable to baseline during AON. This task-related rise in tidal volume paralleled the increase in inspiratory flow rate from NFB to FB to AON conditions. Similarly there was a rise in duty cycle from NFB to AON, suggesting that the most demanding mental performance elicited the greatest changes in central timing and drive mechanisms of respiration, consonant with the largest metabolic effects.

In summary, we found that respiratory adjustments to progressively more demanding mental load followed a pattern by which respiration rate increased to similar levels across all performance condition, whereas incremental elevations of tidal volume--responsive to rather subtle increases in task load and metabolic activity--served to adjust alveolar ventilation so as to accommodate the increased oxygen demand during the most cognitively taxing phases. This pattern of ventilatory adaptation differs from that during exercise, which seems to favor a primary increase in tidal volume, even when adequate levels of ventilation could be easily met by an acceleration of respiration rate (i.e. during isometric handgrip). On the other hand, it is interesting that respiration rate never exceeded about 20 breaths per min for any condition, and it, in fact, remained constant across levels of mental load and dynamic 100-watt exercise. From previous work, it is clear that under greater exertion or other extreme states of physical or emotional distress, respiratory frequency is capable of rising higher. Perhaps, the consistent upper limit we found reflects a physiological ceiling effect under sub-maximal circumstances, so that the human respiratory system operates most optimally or comfortably at or below this upper range.

The foregoing three investigations each explored respiratory adjustments to very repetitive mental tasks essentially paced by exogenous and rapid presentation of visual stimuli. The next study compares effects of two other psychological tasks, one similar to the previous ones with respect to its repetitive and externally paced nature, and the other a task characterized by self-organized mental preparation and anticipation of a immediately subsequent stressful presentation.

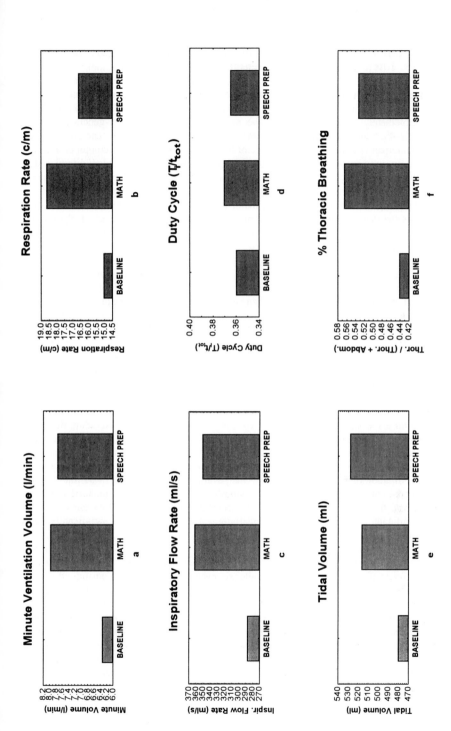

Figure 5. **Respiratory parameters in Study 4: Mean levels during baseline, mental arithmetic and speech preparation.**

Study 4: Computerized Mental Arithmetic *Vs.* Silent Speech Preparation: Externally Vs. Internally Structured Mental Performance

This study investigated respiratory responses to (1) a computer-presented, paced mental arithmetic task, and (2) a condition whereby subjects were required silently to prepare a structured speech that they would immediately thereafter present. The math task was a computer-generated single-, double- and triple-digit addition task with problems presented on a video display, and answers were typed in on a numerical keypad (4 min). The pace of the task was automatically computer-adjusted, so that as performance improved, the length of time permitted for solving a problem diminished. A gift bonus of the equivalent of $50 was offered as a prize for good performance. Prior to the speech preparation task, subjects were presented with an emotionally upsetting scenario (falsely being accused of shoplifting by a security guard in a major department store) and provided with a sheet listing six points that they should address concerning how they might respond and feel in such a situation; they were then told to silently prepare their speech (4 min). Sixty-four adults (21-70 years old) participated.

Figures 5a-f illustrate the respiratory differences between the two task conditions. Minute ventilation volume increased from baseline to both tasks, but did not differ between math performance and speech preparation. In fact, when adjustment was made for dead-space ventilation (based on task variations in respiration rate), alveolar ventilation was almost identical across tasks, indicating that increases in metabolic activity were comparable. Nevertheless, despite this apparent similarity in metabolic demand across tasks, the breathing parameters underlying adjustments in minute ventilation differed. Respiration rate not only increased from baseline to both tasks, but differed between tasks as well, math performance showing the same rapid respiratory frequency previously seen with other repetitive, externally paced tasks (i.e. the MCT and SILT conditions of Studies 1-3). Tidal volume did not increase significantly from baseline to arithmetic performance but did increase during speech preparation. Furthermore, careful examination of the respiratory pattern showed no evidence that subjects displayed sub-vocal speech activity, excluding this factor as a potential source of influence on the breathing pattern (also supported by the absence of duty-cycle differences between baseline and speech preparation). Duty cycle also tended to increase from baseline to math (p <.08), as it generally did in response to the other repetitive externally paced mental tasks. An additional measure that we had available in this study was the thoracic contribution to tidal volume [calculated as ribcage contribution/(ribcage and abdominal)], a measure that can be derived from calibrated Respitrace measurement of tidal volume. With this parameter, we saw a significant increase in thoracic breathing for both tasks, but significantly more pronounced during speech preparation.

Results from this investigation revealed that distinctive breathing patterns mediate ventilatory responses to different types of psychological challenge, even when metabolic demands of the two tasks were apparently equivalent. Math performance, in contrast to baseline, elicited a pronounced thoracic mode of breathing, markedly increased respiration rate and a small rise in duty cycle, with unaltered tidal volume. On the other hand, silent planning for a speech was characterized by more moderate increases in respiration rate and thoracic breathing, as well as a clear elevation in tidal volume and no change in duty cycle, relative to baseline levels. These findings, together with the previously reviewed data, seem to point to a possible difference to respiratory regulation during mental tasks that are internally organized and those that are repetitive and externally paced.

Conclusions

Table 1 provides an overview of the respiratory changes characteristic of the various tasks reviewed above. It should be apparent that no two mental or physical demands elicited precisely the same respiratory pattern. These data suggest a specificity of respiratory responses to mental and physical

Table 1. A summary of respiratory parameter adjustments to distinct mental and physical demands

VARIABLE	Repetitive Mental Task (Moderate)	Repetitive Mental Task (Difficult)	Repetitive Mental Task (Very Difficult)	Quiet Mental Preparation	Isometric Exercise	Aerobic Exercise
Minute Ventilation	↑	↑	↑	↑	↑	↑
Inspiratory Flow	↑	↑	↑	↑	↑	↑
Tidal Volume	↓	↓	=	↑	↑	↑
Respiration Rate	↑	↑	↑	↑	=	↑
Duty Cycle	=	=	↑	=	=	↑

loads that cannot be merely explained by physical energy requirements of the different tasks: Increase in metabolic activity was often similar across active conditions, but a myriad of respiratory adjustments was also evident, which distinguished types of task from each other, as well as even the level of performance within a particular type of task (when motivation was used to alter quality of performance). The major question remains, why does respiratory pattern respond so variably to mental and physical demands even under metabolically equivalent conditions among tasks? We believe that the accommodations to repetitive mental stress must reflect some biological functionality. In other words, there ought to be some adaptive benefit conferred by the breath adjusting the way it does under different psychological and physical demands, unrelated or only loosely related to ventilation's role in metabolic exchange of gases. Confirmatory evidence regarding the adaptive significance of non-metabolically related respiratory adjustments to varieties of behavioral and psychological experience remains unfortunately unavailable. Such knowledge may help us to illuminate the obviously present relations between breathing and emotion in both health and disease [3]. Therefore, we can only propose several plausible hypotheses: Particularly during repetitive, paced mental performance, respiration rate appears to play a primary role in achieving levels of ventilation necessary to meet metabolic requirements. Perhaps, (1) rate can more quickly and efficiently titrate to the relatively subtle, but rapid changes in energy demand of mental tasks; sudden increases in respiration rate will alter alveolar ventilation more quickly than tidal volume changes at constant frequency of breathing. (2) Rate, as opposed to tidal volume, changes, may produce more comfortable and less perceptible sensations of breathing and may, therefore, not interfere as much with conscious performance of certain mental activities. (3) The elevated general muscle tension produced by mental concentration may constrict chest and abdominal muscles so that respiratory rate alterations are easier to make than volume changes. (4) External pacing of mental processes may be more compatible with changes of rate *vs.* volume; both task and physiological process, in this case, are bound together as a function of time. (5) Finally, changes in rate and/or volume may be secondary to central, generalized arousal patterns which may have other primary adaptive purposes, so that respiratory adjustments beyond those necessary to meet metabolic demands may be epiphenomenal. These are, of course, just some of the possibilities that might explain why breathing changes as it does to varieties of behavioral experience. In this brief review of our finding, we have attempted a primarily descriptive analysis of how breathing patterns vary to certain psychological and physical demands. We hope that research may start to address the question of why breathing changes as it does during different behavioral states.

References

1. Pine DS, Coplan JD, Papp LA, Klein RG, Martinez JM, Kovalenko P (1998) Ventilatory physiology of children and adolescents with anxiety disorders. *Arch Gen Psychiat* 55:123-129
2. Roth WT, Wilhelm FH, Trabert W (1998) Voluntary breath holding in panic and generalized anxiety disorders. *Psychosom Med* 60:671-679
3. Grossman P(1983) Respiration, stress and cardiovascular function. *Psychophysiol* 20:284-300
4. Grossman P, Wientjes,CJ (1989) Respiratory Disorders: Asthma and Hyperventilation Syndrome. In: Turpin G (ed) *Handbook of Clinical Psychophysiology*. New York: Wiley, pp 519-554
5. Wientjes C, Grossman P, Gaillard A, Defares P (1986) Individual differences in respiration and stress. In: Hockey GR, Gaillard A, Coles MG (eds) *Energetics and information processing*. Dordrecht (the Netherlands): Martinus Nijhoff pp 317-327
6. Wientjes CJ, Grossman P, Gaillard, A (1998)Influence of drive and timing mechanisms on breathing pattern and ventilation during mental performance. *Biological Psychology* 49:53-70
7. Wientjes CJ, Grossman P (1994) Overreactivity of the psyche or the soma? Interindividual associations between psychosomatic symptoms, anxiety, heart rate, and end-tidal partial carbon dioxide pressure. *Psychosom Med* 56:533-40
8. Wientjes CJ (1993) *Psychological Influences upon Breathing: Situational and Dispositional Aspects*. The Hague: CIP-Data Koninklijke Bibliotheek

Anxiety and Respiration

Yuri Masaoka, Arata Kanamaru and Ikuo Homma

Second Department of Physiology, Showa University School of Medicine, 1-5-8 Hatanodai, Tokyo 142-8555, Japan

Summary: Recent research on emotions has been investigated by neuropsychologists using PET and fMRI. The location of neuronal activity during production of emotions such as happiness, sad, fear and anxiety in the human brain is becoming clear. However, emotional experiences are not only productions within the brain accompanied by physiological activity such as sweating, increasing heart rate and respiration; these activities result from an unconscious process. Respiration, one of the physiological activities, is also expressed unconsciously. The activities of breathing in and breathing out are a curious mechanism because this activity comes from the unconscious regulation of a metabolic requirement, and simultaneously expresses emotion involuntarily. In this chapter, we compare the effect of physical load and mental stress tests on metabolic outputs and respiratory timing, and demonstrate the effect of both emotional states. The results indicate that there is a correlation between anxiety levels and respiratory rate: the increase of minute ventilation involves individual anxiety. We also provide evidence that anticipatory anxiety increases respiratory rate without metabolic change and during this time dipoles are concentrated in the paralimbic area temporal pole estimated by the dipole tracing method. From our results, we discuss the relation between respiration and emotion of anxiety from psychological and physiological view points.

Key words: Physical load, Mental stress, Emotion, Anxiety, Respiratory rate, Dipole tracing method, Paralimbic area

RESPIRATORY OUTPUTS FROM METABOLISM AND HIGHER CENTER

In the human brain, two neural systems control respiration. One system originates in the pons and the medulla, controlling respiratory muscles by descending impulses through the spinal cord to the motor neurons. The other system, voluntary control originates in cerebral the cortex. This voluntary or behavioral control system interrupts the autonomic control breathing system, for example, during speech. In an awake state, the respiratory pattern comes from a complex interaction between matching for a metabolic requirement and a non-metabolic demand, such as arousal level and sensory stimulation (1). The non metabolic factor also includes emotions. Many studies have demonstrated that emotions such as fear, unpleasantness, joy, happiness, etc., affect respiratory activity (2). These data made clear that respiratory activity is related to emotions which are from the limbic area.

The first study made clear how respiratory activity interacts between regulation for the metabolic demand and information from the higher center.   To compare the differences of the center output of respiration between two factors, we analyzed the respiratory pattern and the metabolic outputs during an isometric leg exercise (physical load test) and a mental stress test (3).   The physical load test was produced by attaching a Velcro belt with a spring balance wrapped around the subjects' knees and the subjects were asked to stretch their knees in an outer direction, holding a 7-Kg load.   For the mental stress test, subjects wore a headphone to deliver noxious sounds with a volume set at 73dbA.   We also measured the emotional state (unpleasantness or difficulty of task) during tests and anxiety levels in order to determine the relationship between these psychological factors and respiration.   On a breath-by-breath basis, we measured the subjects' minute ventilation (V_E), tidal volume (V_T), respiratory rate (RR), O_2 consumption (VO_2), CO_2 production (VCO_2) and end-tidal fraction of CO_2 (F_{ETCO2}) with an aeromoniter AE280.   Our hypothesis was that respiratory pattern would correlate with the level of unpleasantness and difficulty of task. The study found that there was no correlation between the level of emotional state and the respiratory parameters in both tests, but there was a positive significant correlation between anxiety scores and respiratory rate (Figure1).   People with high state anxiety showed an increase in RR during the physical load test, and people with high trait anxiety showed an increase in RR during the mental stress test.   On the basis of this study, we investigated the metabolic outputs during both tests and analyzed the respiratory timing relationship between inspiration and expiration, taking into account individual anxiety level.

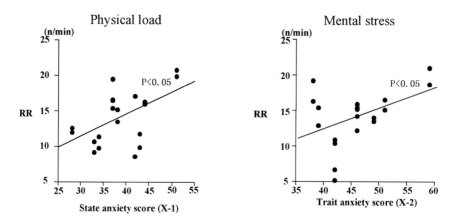

Fig.1. Correlation between respiratory rate (RR) and state anxiety scores during physical load (left), and between RR and trait anxiety scores during metal stress (right).   Data derived from Reference (3).

THE EFFECT OF INDIVIDUAL ANXIETY LEVEL ON EXPIRATORY TIME

In this study, breath-by-breath metabolic outputs during physical load were compared with the outputs during noxious audio stimulation (4). The protocol and the level of stimulation used were the same as the preceding study. Disregarding anxiety level, there was a linear relationship between V_E and VO_2 during the physical load (Figure 2, left). On the other hand, during the mental stress there was no linear relationship between V_E and VO_2 (Figure 2, right). This increase of V_E was not to meet a metabolic requirement. In the physical load test, an increase of V_E appeared not only to meet the metabolic need but also to include the non-metabolic need, indicating an increase of V_E/VO_2 ratio in the group with high anxiety (Table 1).

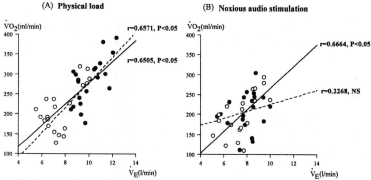

Fig. 2. Plots of minute ventilation (V_E) and O_2 consumption (VO_2) during baseline ($\bigcirc$ with solid line) and during physical load and mental stress ($\bullet$ with dotted line). Data derived from Reference (4).

Table 1. (A) Effects of physical load on V_E/VO_2 for subjects with low and with high state anxiety.
(B) Effects of noxious audio stimulation on V_E/VO_2 for subjects with low and with high trait anxiety.
Values indicate mean $\pm$ SD. Statistical difference from control, **:P<0.001, **P<0.01, *P<0.05. Data derived from Reference (4).

(A)

	Subjects with low state anxiety		Subjects with high state anxiety	
	Baseline	Load	Baseline	Load
V_E/VO_2	0.039 ± 0.010	$0.038\pm0.017*$	0.036 ± 0.009	$0.046\pm0.086***$
V_E/VCO_2	0.041 ± 0.009	$0.042\pm0.042***$	0.041 ± 0.009	$0.043\pm0.046***$

(B)

	Subjects with low trait anxiety		Subjects with high trait anxiety	
	Baseline	Noxious audio stim.	Baseline	Noxious audio stim.
V_E/VO_2	0.036 ± 0.008	$0.035\pm0.009*$	0.038 ± 0.011	$0.052\pm0.072*$
V_E/VCO_2	0.04 ± 0.006	$0.037\pm0.007***$	0.041 ± 0.01	$0.046\pm0.056*$

Values indicate mean $\pm$ SD
Statistical difference from control, ***P<0.001, **P<0.01, *P<0.05.

58

In both tests, correlation between VO_2 and anxiety level was not observed. These data also suggest that V_E is related not only to fulfillment of the metabolic demand but also to anxiety which is associated with RR. From an analysis of the respiratory timing relationship concerning the increase of RR, there was a negative correlation between the decrease in T_E and anxiety in both tests. Based on these data, we made a diagram illustrating a possible mechanism of the V_T-T_E relationship, which accounted for each individual (Figure 3). The study suggests that in an awake state anxiety may dominantly affect the RR, especially on the T_E.

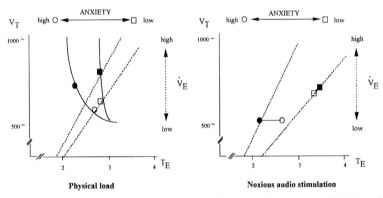

Figure 3. Diagrams illustrating possible mechanism of V_T-T_E, taking into account individual anxiety levels. Data derived from Reference (4).

WHAT IS ANXIETY?

In these studies, respiratory rate always correlated with the individual anxiety scores. So the question is, what is anxiety? According to a psychological definition of anxiety (5), anxiety is described as "the tense anticipation of a threatening but vague event; a feeling of uneasy suspense." Anxiety is distinguished from fear (Table 2). Fear has a specific focus and is from the outside world; people can understand the connection between threat and fear. Fear recedes or ceases when danger is removed. Fear, according to Joseph LeDoux (6) "is related to the behavioral acts of escape and avoidance in threatening situations, and when these actions are thwarted, fear becomes anxiety." Anxiety is regarded as a negative feeling and people always think it is important to reduce anxiety. However, anxiety play an important role in human life because if we don't have anxiety, we can not avoid dangerous situations; we could not even take out disaster insurance! Anxiety is one of the human core emotional feelings which helps us defend ourselves.

Table 2. Differences between fear and anxiety.   Data derived from Reference (5).

Fear	Anxiety
Specific focus of threat	Source of threat is elusive
Understandable connection	Uncertain connection between
between threat and fear	anxiety and threat
Usually episodic	Prolonged
Circumscribed tension	Pervasive uneasiness
Identifiable threat	Can be objectless
Provoked by threat cues	Uncertain onset
Declines with removal of threat	Persistent
Offset is detectable	Uncertain offset
Circumscribed area of threat	Without clear borders
Imminent threat	Threat seldom imminent
Quality of an emergency	Heightened vigilance
Bodily sensations of an emergency	Bodily sensations of vigilance
Rational quality	Puzzling quality

ANTICIPATORY ANXIETY

Studies so far have investigated the effect of mental stress and physical load on respiratory parameters, and the effect of these tests involved individual anxiety trait, which is associated with RR.   Subsequently, we focused on the effect of anxiety itself on respiratory patterns and metabolic outputs by creating a situation that produced anxiety in the subjects.   The hypothesis was that if an increase of RR was affected by emotion of anxiety in the brain, the metabolic increase and cardiac activity would remain unchanged.   If so, what was the relationship between trait anxiety scores and respiratory pattern.   Anxiety was produced from an external danger by attaching electrical stimulation (ES) to the left forefinger.   The subjects were informed that ES would be delivered sometime within two minutes after the warning red light (WRL) which was installed 1.5m from the subject's head.   All subjects' anxiety levels were tested by STAI (Spielberger's State Trait Anxiety); during the experiment their anxiety levels were measured by Visual Analogue Scale(VAS).   The subjects reported that the ES was not painful but they were anxious about the impending ES after seeing the WRL.   Anxiety produced in this study is called "anticipatory anxiety."   Anticipatory anxiety is often observed in patients with panic disorder and anxiety disorder because the attack is not be predictable and not related to any situation or stimulation.

Ten subjects were studied.   This study found that V_E increased unchanged VO_2, VCO_2 and heart rate (HR).   The subjects with high trait anxiety showed an increase in RR.   Tobin et al. have shown that the mere anticipation of exercise causes an increase in ventilation and emphasize the importance of cortical factors (7).   From our data, there is no doubt that a mechanism of enhancement of respiratory output exists in the higher structure; this increase of RR is not for meeting the metabolic need nor homeostatic purpose.

RESPIRATORY-RELATED ANXITY POTENTIAL (RAP) IN THE HUMAN BRAIN

It has been reported in an animal study that electrical stimulation of a higher center such as the amygdala and temporal pole alters the breathing pattern (8, 9), and a human study shows the role of the amygdala in anxiety (10). Recent research on neuronal activity in the human brain has been carried out using positron emission tomography (PET) and fMRI. These studies have made clear the neuroanatomical correlation of various emotions. However, a study concerning the neurological correlation of physiological changes during the production of emotion has not been investigated. Emotions, we feel, occur with physiological responses; feedback is needed for the emotional experience (6).

We used the dipole tracing method (DT method) of a skull-scalp-brain (SSB) head model (DT/SSB) (as described in Dr. Homma's chapter) (11, 12) to determine the electric current sources during the production of anticipatory anxiety (13). The advantage of this method is that potentials which recorded from 21 electrodes are able to average as a trigger of physiological response such as sweating and respiration. The averaged potentials were analyzed by DT/SSB.

Our hypothesis is that if the subjective feeling of anxiety enhances the respiratory rate, the electric current sources synchronized with this onset of inspiration could be found somewhere in the higher structure. Anticipatory anxiety was produced by electrical stimulation which indicated "Anticipatory anxiety." The onset of inspiration taken during anticipation of electrical shock was used as the trigger of the EEG. Figure 4 indicates the level of anxiety and respiratory rate increases during anticipation of electrical shock.

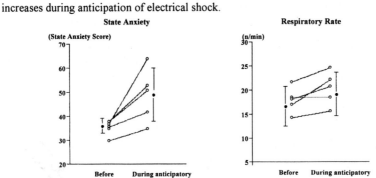

Fig. 4. State anxiety scores (left) and respiratory rate (right) before the warning red light and during anticipation of electrical stimuli for 5 subjects. Significant differences between the two conditions were observed (left; Wilcoxson Signed Rank Test, P<0.05., right; Repeated Measurement ANOVA, P<0.05).

EEG were averaged by the onset of the inspiration of this increased respiratory rate. From 350ms to 400ms after the onset of inspiration, a positive wave was observed in three subjects. These positive waves were observed in people with high trait anxiety: this wave is referred to as Respiratory-related Anxiety Potential (RAP). Results of DT/SSB, electric current sources were found in the right temporal pole (Figure 5). Neural activity during anticipatory anxiety, we found, was synchronized with the onset of inspiration. These areas were the same as Reiman's anticipatory anxiety research made by PET (14). According to Reiman, the temporal pole referred to as the "paralimbic area", could play the role of evaluating and characterizing a situation with uncertainty and danger.

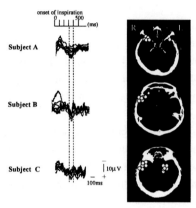

Fig. 5. Respiratory- related Anxiety Potentials (RAP) in three subjects. White circles highlight the areas in which the number of dipoles are concentrated the most in each head model. Data derived from Reference (13).

CONCLUSION

1. In the physical load and the mental stress tests, there was no correlation between the emotional score levels and the respiratory parameters, but there was a positive correlation between respiratory rate and anxiety level.
2. Analysis of VO_2 and anxiety levels showed no correlation. V_E increased not only to meet the metabolic demand but also to include a factor from the higher center; anxiety participates in this increase, and in particular, anxiety affected on T_E.
3. An increase of respiratory rate is associated with anticipatory anxiety, and that during this time electric current sources were observed in the temporal pole; these neural activities were synchronized with the onset of inspiration.

ANXIETY AND RESPIRATORY RATE THE QUESTION IS WHICH OCCURS FIRST?

During the feeling of anticipatory anxiety, both respiratory rate and anxiety state increased. This increase of respiratory rate was not caused by an increase of metabolism, and the subjects did not inspire voluntarily. Neural activity in the temporal pole was synchronized with the onset of inspiration of an unconscious increase of respiratory rate. However, if anxiety enhances the respiratory rate, the source must be found before the onset of inspiration. Our results indicated that dipoles were concentrated in the temporal pole from 350ms to 400 ms after the onset of inspiration. If the temporal pole is regarded as "feeling of anxiety related area", would this area have been activated before the onset of inspiration?

DOES ANXIETY ENHANCE THE RESPIRATORY RATE OR DOES RESPIRATORY RATE PRODUCE ANXIETY?

This question reminds us of the debates between the James-Lang and Cannon-Bird theory; the two theories of emotion question whether feelings cause emotional responses or responses cause feelings. From our data, it may be hypothesized that respiratory rate immediately increases before we are aware of the emotional feeling of anxiety. Stimulus from the outside world transmit through the sensory thalamus to certain places in the brain which evaluate whether the target is dangerous or safe (Schema 1). During evaluation of the target, respiratory rate immediately increases. An increase of respiratory rate produces more anxiety; therefore, the level of anxiety may result from the number of times the person inspires. A feeling of anxiety also produces an adverse effect on increase of respiratory rate. The level of conscious state of anxiety may be determined by this multiplier effect produced by the circuit between anxiety and respiratory rate.

LeDoux (6) indicated in the studies on conditioned emotional responses in fear that information of external stimuli reaches the amygdala directly by the pathway from the thalamus, bypassing the sensory cortex. The conditioning process affects breathing (7, 15) and our study shows that an increase of respiratory rate observed in anticipation of electrical stimulation, especially in people with high trait anxiety may involve the mechanism of conditioning. It could be said that production of anxiety associated with an increase of respiratory rate may include the capacity of the individual's defense mechanism.

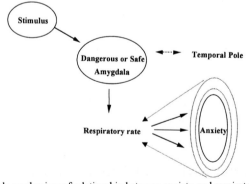

Schema 1   Possible mechanism of relationship between anxiety and respiratory rate.

Two questions remain unanswered. One is why does respiratory rate increase in people with anxiety? Is there any advantage of this increase; for example, can we run away faster or can sense a dangerous situation? The other is if we voluntarily breathe slowly, is anxiety modified? The respiratory control system is complicated but it is a curious system because we can control ourselves; we can consciously breath in and slowly because of the cortical area. Does our intention dominate the control of anxiety? The unsolved mechanism is in the respiratory control system and these question must be clarified in our future research.

REFERENCES

1. Shea SA (1996) Behavioral and arousal-related influences on breathing in humans. Experimental Physiology 81:1-26

2. Boiten FA, Frijda NH, Wientjes CJE (1994) Emotions and respiratory pattern: review and critical analysis. International Journal of Psychophysiology 17:103-128

3. Masaoka Y, Homma I (1997) Anxiety and respiratory patterns: their relationship during mental stress and physical load. International Journal of Psychophysiology 27:153-159

4. Masaoka Y, Homma I (1999) Expiratory time determined by individual anxiety levels in humans Journal Applied Physiology 86(4):1329-1336

5. Rachaman S (1998) Anxiety. Psychology Press LTD, East Sussex.

6. Joseph L (1999) The emotional Brain, Phoenix, London

7. Tobin MJ, Perez W, Guenther SM, D'Alonzo G, Dantzker DR (1986) Breathing pattern and metabolic behavior during anticipation of exercise. Journal Applied Physiology 60(4):1306-1312

8. Kaada BR, Pribram KH, Epstein JA (1949) Respiratory and vascular responses in monkeys from temporal pole, insula, orbital surface and cingulate gyrus. Journal Neurophysiology 12:348-356

9. Harper, R. M., Frysinger, R. C., Trelease, R. B. and Marks, J.D., State-dependent alternation of respiratory cycle timing by stimulation of the central nucleus of the amygdala (1984) Brain Research 306:1-8

10. Davis, M The role of the amygdala in fear and anxiety (1992) Annual Review Neuroscience 15:353-375

64

11. Homma S, Musha T, Nakajima Y, Okamoto Y, Blom S, Flink R, Hagbarth K.E (1995) Conductivity ratios of the scalp-skull-brain head model in estimating equivalent dipole sources in human brain. Neuroscience Research 22:51-55

12. Kanamaru A, Homma I, Hara T (1999) Movement related cortical sources for elbow flexion in patients with brachial plexus injury after intercostal-musculocutaneous nerve crossing,. Neuroscience Letter 274:203-206

13. Masaoka Y, Homma I (2000) The source generator of Respiratory-related Anxiety Potential (RAP) in the human brain. Neuroscience Letter 283: 21-24

14. Reiman EM, Fusselman MJ, Fox PT, Raichle ME (1989) Neuroanatomical correlates of anticiatory anxiety. Science 243:1071-1074

15. Gallego J, Perruchet P (1991) Classical conditioning of ventilatory responses in humans. Journal Applied Physiology 70 (2): 676-682

Respiration and the Emotion of Dyspnea/Suffocation Fear

Ronald Ley

University at Albany, State University of New York
228 Ed Bldg. 1400 Washington Ave., Albany, NY 12222, USA

Summary: The thesis of this paper is that the experience of acute severe dyspnea accompanied by dyspnea/suffocation fear are prerequisites for the classic primary panic attack (1, 2). The probability that the occurrence of a single panic attack leads to panic disorder depends on the intensity and duration of the initial attack and whether or not the accompanying environmental cues (endogenous and/or exogenous) facilitate generalization of dyspnea/suffocation fear to a relatively broad range of stimuli. Thus, an initial classic panic attack is less likely to lead to subsequent secondary panic attacks (attacks of dyspnea/suffocation fear in the absence of severe dyspna) or to tertiary attacks (relatively mild anxiety/apprehension elicited by anticipatory thoughts, and their antecedents, of prior primary or secondary attacks) if the initial primary attack occurs in a relatively unique environment.

This dyspnea/suffocation fear theory of panic is based on information derived from clinical self reports, surveys, controlled studies, analyses of adventitious panic attacks (2, 3, 4, 5, 6, 7, 8), principles of respiratory physiology, and essays on the biological nature of fear as an adaptive response. The purpose of this paper is to review research on relevant issues of respiratory psychophysiology as they pertain to the thesis that stress-induced dyspnea with concomitant dyspnea/suffocation fear, especially hyperventilation stress-induced dyspnea, underlie (a) primary panic attacks, (b) the Pavlovian/classical conditioning of dyspnea/suffocation fear in secondary panic attacks, and (c) the anxious apprehension that characterizes the discomfort of the tertiary panic attack. (2).

DYSPNEA/SUFFOCATION FEAR THEORY OF PANIC DISORDER

The tripartite classification of panic attacks proposed by Ley (2) was an outgrowth of clinical reports and laboratory controlled studies of panic attacks which pointed to the centrality of unsignaled tachycardia and seemingly uncontrollable dyspnea, i.e., uncontrollable in terms of a sense of loss of self-regulation of breathing like that experienced when one's "wind is knocked out." The emotion that accompanies the primary (Type I) panic attack during this brief period of respiratory retardation, a period during which voluntary effort will initiate satisfactory breathing, is referred to here as dyspnea/suffocation fear. In terms of a Pavlovian conditioning paradigm, the dyspnea and dyspnea/suffocation fear can be conceptualized as an unconditioned response (UCR) complex composed of dyspnea with dyspnea/suffocation fear as the emotional component of the complex. The hyperventilation related physical/psychological antecedents of dyspnea would constitute the unconditional stimulus (UCS) –see below.

The secondary (Type II) panic attack was postulated as a conditioned response (CR), i.e., dyspnea/suffocation fear, the emotional component of the UCR elicited by events (exogenous and/or endogenous) associated with the occasion of the UCR. Tertiary (Type III) panic attacks constitute a category of self reports of symptoms that meet the DSM IV criteria for inclusion in the classification of panic but which present with few or no physiologically discernible autonomic responses comparable to those presented in cases of type I or Type II attacks. Patients classified as sufferers of Type III panic attacks also present with less florid accounts of onset of symptoms. The issue of "types" of panic attacks is reviewed here because the results of studies of panic cannot be compared if the crucial issue of whether or not the phenomenon in question is the same from study to study.

BIOLOGICAL PRIMACY OF BREATHING

Breathing leads the list of vital needs in terms of the limits of time of deprivation; without an adequate supply of oxygen (O2) cells die within minutes and life ends. The experience that signals the imminence of lethal suffocation is dyspnea. Perhaps the earliest psychophysiological analysis of the occurrences of hyperventilation, dyspnea, and dyspnea/suffocation fear, that mark the classic panic attack reported by a scientist was that of William James (9):

> ...if inability to draw deep breath, fluttering of the heart, and that peculiar epigastric change felt as "precordial anxiety,"...and with perhaps other visceral processes not now known, all spontaneously occur together in a certain person, his feeling of their combination is the emotion of dread, and he is the victim of what is known as morbid fear. A friend who has had occasional attacks of this most distressing of all maladies tells me that in his case the whole drama seems to centre about the regions of the heart and respiratory apparatus, that his main effort during the attacks is to get control of his inspiration and to slow down his heart, and that the moment he attains to breathing deeply and to holding himself erect, the dread, ipso facto, seems to depart (pp.244-245).

The claim that panic with dyspnea/suffocation fear is the "most distressing of all maladies" has been corroborated more recently by Aiken, Zeally, and Rosenthal (10): "Dyspnea may be felt as endagering to life to a greater extent than almost any other symptom: to the patient, the experience of dyspnea is regarded as something which, if it worsens to asphyxia, must be fatal" (p. 256). Although dyspnea is like pain insofar as it often is accompanied by the emotionally adaptive experience of fear, it has received relatively little attention as a psychophysiological construct that may play a central role in panic disorder and other respiratory-related psychosomatic complains (11, 12). Part of the reason for this may lie in difficulties inherent to a scientific analysis of psychophysiological constructs, such as dyspnea, that depend on the methods of psychophysics for their measurement.

The possible routes from the physical antecedents of dyspnea to the sensation of dyspnea are very complex; they involve afferent impulses from pulmonary sensory receptors that are relayed via vagal and sympathetic pathways, afferent impulses from muscular receptors that are transmitted to the central nervous system, central collateral discharge (interneurons in the CNS that transduce intensity of output to muscles), receptors in the upper airways including the nose and larynx, and chemoreceptors that respond to hypoxia, hypercapnia, and changes in hydrogen ion concentration. If pressed to give my best guess, I would posit that dyspnea is a consequence of a multi-factor interaction in which muscular receptors and chemoreceptors play key roles with muscular receptors front stage and chemoreceptors backstage. The reason I suspect that muscular receptors are primary is because they are immediately responsible for breathing, i.e., moving air in and out of the lungs. This also suggests possible involvement of the phrenic nerve, which, if short-circuited, might produce the acute paralysis that marks having ones "wind knocked out," as well as contribute to the dyspnea that marks the Type I panic attack. Research findings on this issue are mixed. Most important for the purpose of the present paper is that there are several possible routes to dyspnea.

PULMONARY FUNCTION AND HYPERVENTILATION

Although both hypoventilation (underbreathing) and hyperventilation (overbreathing) that exceed the bounds of typical variations in ventilation called for by the requirements of day-to-day living can have effects on the sense of dyspnea as well as cognitive processs, the effects of hyperventilation are of greater psychological interest, effects of blood pH aside, because their induction can be the consequence of both voluntarily and reflexive overbreathing elicited by emotional arousal and sympathetic nervous system excitation. Voluntary hypoventilation, on the other hand, can be induced by breathholding only for relatively brief periods of time limited by the build up of CO_2 which will stimulated the respiratory centers and thereby induce resumption of breathing. Thus, hyperventilation and its immediate effects on pH, especially as it affects cerebral oxygenation (hypoxia) and cardiovascular function (ischemia), has been the focus of research in respiratory-related psychophysiological complaints. Other active researchers in the fields of panic disorder acknowledge the salience of hyperventilation in the diagnosis and treatment prognosis of panic. In the abstract of a recent paper, Papp, Coplan, Klein, Woods, Shear, Barlow, and Gorman (13) state that:

> One of the most consistently reported respiratory abnormalities in patients with panic disorder is the tendency to hyperventilate. If hyperventilation induced low end-tidal CO_2 level is a state specific phenomenon, clinical remission, regardless of treatment modality, should normalize ETCO2....ETCO2 is a convenient respiratory parameter that can be easily utilized to predict and monitor treatment response in a least a subgroup of patients with panic disorder.

The basic significance of pulmonary function and dyspnea in panic disorder has also been emphasized by Klein (14) in his "false suffocation alarm" theory. However, unlike Ley's (15) dyspnea/suffocation theory, Klein alludes to dyspnea only indirectly in his reference to a hypothetical "deranged suffocation monitor" which is claimed to trigger a maladaptive hypothetical "suffocation alarm," that alerts the suffer that there is a lack of useful air. One problem with the theory is that is does not account for common cases of suffocation/asphyxia in which people die but experience no apparent alarm (e.g., carbon monoxide poisoning, prolonged inhalation of nitrogen, sleep apnea). Another problem is that the theory cannot account for Fowler's (16) findings that the latency of breath holding can be increased significantly with inhalations of air enriched with 7.5% and 8.2% CO_2, gases which increase arterial CO_2 beyond the 5% CO_2 level used in Klein's challenge test which purportedly fires the putative "suffocation alarm." (17).

Perhaps most important, Klein does not address the distinction between "dyspnea" and "suffocation," namely, that dyspnea refers to the sense that breathing is impaired, whereas "suffocation" refers to the condition of impeded breathing. Thus dyspnea will be experienced if suffocation occurs as a result of bronchial constriction in asthma, but dyspnea will not be experienced if suffocation occurs as the result of anoxia caused by prolonged inhalation of carbon monoxide (CO). The distinction between "dyspnea" and "suffocation" is essential for the purpose of comparison and evaluation of theories (18).

In a study designed to test a hypothesis derived from dyspnea/suffocation theory, Asmundson and Stein (19) reasoned that the severity of panic disorder (a function of dyspnea/suffocation fear) might be correlated with pulmonary function. Since dyspnea is a symptom of pulmonary dysfunction and since forced expiratory flow rate (FEF) is used in the detection of obstructive airway disease, the index of pulmonary function they chose to measure was FEF 50%, the rate of expiratory air flow in L/min at the moment when vital capacity is half (50%) the volume present at the onset of expiration.

To test the hypothesis that panic-disorder patients may suffer diminished lung function, Asmundson and Stein subjected 15 panic patients to a lung function test in which they measured forced expiratory volume during the first second of expiration (FEV1) and forced vital capacity. Since expiratory flow rate is a negatively decelerating function of expiratory time, maximal expiratory flow rate occurs at the beginning of expiration. Thus the mid-region of the expiratory flow curve provides a measure of flow rate that is most sensitive to detection of airway obstructions which might be symptomatic of pulmonary disease and the severity of a sense of dyspnea, i.e., flow rate is positively correlated with healthy pulmonary function.

Based on the lung function test, patients were divided into two groups: the eight with the slowest expiratory flow rate were designated as "Low FEF 50% PD patients" and the seven with the fastest rates were designed "High FEF 50% PD patients." Consistent with predictions based on the dyspnea/suffocation fear theory, the Low FEF 50% PD patients had higher scores than the High FEF 50% PD patients on all eight self-report measures of panic severity, five of which were statistically significant (state anxiety, % endorsed symptoms from Anxiety Symptom Questionnaire, global symptom severity, respiratory symptoms, and cognitive/fear symptoms). (For a detailed discussion, see Ley (15).

CONDITIONED VENTILATION AND DYSPNEA/SUFFOCATION FEAR

Although the findings of Asmundson and Stein (19) suggest that the propensity to panic disorder may be a function of compromised pulmonary function, a relatively broad range of changes in ventilatory behavior (e.g., respiration frequency, respiration volume, pattern of breathing, apneic pauses) can be modified in humans and a variety of other animals; and dyspnea/suffocation fear as an acquired emotion appears to be readily conditioned in animals and healthy patients with no history of panic attacks. (For a recent survey, 6).

Research on escape and avoidance behavior has in the main used electric shock or conditioned fear as noxious motivational states. None the less, there have been a few studies that have employed aversive ventilatory states (dyspnea) as a source of motivation. Broadhurst (20) submerged rats in water and required them to learn to discriminate between the brighter of two sides of an underwater maze in order to escape. Several levels of difficulty in the discrimination problem were studied in conjunction with five different intervals of submersion (0, 2, 4, 6, or 8 sec) prior to release in the maze. Broadhurst found that performance in the maze was a function of level of air deprivation. Thus, levels of presumed dyspnea/suffocation fear (time of air deprivation before release in the maze) motivated behavior in a manner parallel to levels of a primary appetitive need (e.g., hunger or thirst) or levels of a primary aversive need (e.g., pain) or levels of strength of an acquired motive (e.g., fear or frustration).

Another study that demonstrated the noxious quality of dyspnea (i.e., air deprivation) was conducted by Leukel abd Quinton (21). After rats were trained to jump a hurdle to escape shock, a subgroup of animals was subjected to CO_2 anesthetization immediately following the hurdle jump. Poor performance on subsequent opportunities to avoid shock indicates the noxious character of breathing large concentrations of coma-inducing CO_2. i.e., the dyspnea/suffocation fear induced by the large concentration of CO_2 overrode fear elicited by the anticipation of shock.

In a controlled experiment with human subjects, Cambell, Sanderson, and Laverty (22) provided dramatic evidence that dyspnea/suffocation fear can be acquired as a CR following a single conditioning trial. Using succinylcholine chloride dihydrate to induce respiratory paralysis (UCS), they paired a tone (CS) with 90- to 100-sec periods of the induced paralysis. On subsequent presentations of the CS following a single conditioning trial, subjects exhibited a complex CR consisting of virtually inexhaustible bouts of increases respiration rate, heart rate, increases electrodermal conductivity, and florid self reports of fear.

Evidence that dyspnea/suffocation fear can be conditioned in a single trial in rats was recently reported by Mongeluzi, Rosellini, Caldarone, Stock and Abrahamsen (23). In this carefully controlled experiment, rats were placed individually in an atmospherically controlled chamber permeated with the odor of vanilla (CS) for a 5-min period, the last 30 sec of which the chamber was infused with 100% CO_2 (UCS). The day following this single conditioning trial, half of the animals were placed in the test chamber containing the odor of vanilla in room air (i.e., CS but no UCS) for an eight-min period during which freezing behavior (inhibition of movement, an index of fear) was measured. The other half of the conditioned group was tested in the absence of the CS; and a third group that had not been conditioned was tested in the presence of the CS. The results pointed clearly to the fear-eliciting potency of the CS in the context of the conditioning chamber for the animals that had received the single conditioning trial on the day prior to testing, an effect that was notably resistant to extinction. These results were replicated in a second experiment (24) in which the intensity of the UCS (concentration of CO_2: 0%, 5%, 35%, 100%) was varied. Animals exposed to 100% CO_2 showed greater resistance to extinction (i.e., a more gradual decrease in magnitude of CR over extinction trials) than animals exposed to 35% CO_2 and 5% CO_2 (no evidence of conditioning in the 0% CO_2 group), results which suggest strongly that the magnitude of the fear conditioning was a direct function of the severity of dyspnea experienced during the single conditioning trial. The data of this animal model lend strong support to the dyspnea/suffocation fear theory of panic disorder.

CONDITIONED RESPIRATORY RESISTANCE

Although the routes between the physiological antecedents of dyspnea and the sensation of dyspnea are complex, the empirical fact that respiratory resistance produces dyspnea is clear. Constriction of the bronchi during an asthma attack produces dyspnea. Putting aside the complexity of the physiological routes to dyspnea, research on Pavlovian conditioning of respiratory resistance and resulting dyspnea is a fascinationg topic that may help to explain how respiratory psychophysiology provides a bridge between the physiological routes of dyspnea and the psychological sensation of dyspnea.

Total respiratory resistance (the impedence in the flow of air through the airways, lung tissue, and chest wall) is an important factor in the maintenance of good health in general and a critical factor in disease, especially chronic lung disease (asthma, bronchitis, and emphysema). Because asthma is so prevalent in the general population, the asthmatic attack (dyspnea evoked by the reduction in breathing that results from insufficient expiration) is commonly understood to be caused by constriction of the bronchioles, i.e. severe increase in total respiratory resistance. While the rudimentary physiology of asthma (involuntary controls of breathing) have been well researched, voluntary control of breathing as a factor in the evocation of asthmatic breathing has received relatively little attention. Several studies that point to the conditionability of airway/respiratory resistance will be noted here.

One of the first studies to the demonstrate that asthma attacks could be acquired as a Pavlovian conditioned response was conducted by Dekker, Pelser and Groen (25). Although an increase in total respiratory resistance is a feature of asthma attacks, the conditionability of increased respiratory resistance need not be limited to asthmatics if an agent other that an asthma-specific allergen can be identified as a UCS for the evocation of an increase in respiratory resistance as the UCR.   Kotses, Westland and Greer (26) identified such an agent, a mental stress test that requires subjects to count backwards by 17s.   Following the procedures of a differential conditioning paradigm, Miller and Kotses (27) paired one of two colored lights with a UCS (counting backwards by 17s) that evoked an increase in total respiratory resistance.   Over the last one of seven conditioning trials, the increase in total respiratory resistance elicited by the CS+ was greater than that elicited by the CS-, i.e., increased total respiratory resistance can be aquired as a CR by means of Pavlovian conditioning.   Given that dyspnea is the sensation that accompanies increased respiratory resistance, these findings have important implications for the diagnosis and treatment of respiratory psychophysiological disorders in general and for Ley's dyspnea/suffocation fear theory of panic attacks in particular.   That is, increased respiratory resistance as a UCR to stress, may account for the unexpected "out-of-the blue" onset of uncontrollable dyspnea and its accompanying dyspneic/suffocation fear, the fear that characterizes the classic type I panic attack (1, 2).

CONDITIONED HYPERVENTILATION

The ubiquitous nature of hyperventilation as a dominant respiratory abnormality in the classic attack (i.e., at least one subgroup of patient with panic disorder) has been well established (13).   However, the implications of the effects of hyperventilation on a broad range of psychosomatic complains beyond panic disorder have been discussed by Lum (28).   In a well reasoned and persuasive essay, Lum (28) has argued that there are "susceptible individuals [who] have required a habit of breathing in such a way that the day-to-day level of arterial CO_2 is low, or that the normal hyperventilatory response to physical or emotional stimului is exaggerated....With frequent repetition, the response takes on the characteristics of a conditioned reflex." (p. 198).

In earlier studies of conditioned breathing in which CRs were defined as increases in respiratory frequency and/or volume conditioned hyperventilation almost certainly occurred; but these studies did not measure PCO_2, a decrement in which defines conditioned hyperventilation. Most recently, however, Ley (29) monitored end-tidal CO_2 (ETCO2) continuously in healthy adults throughout all phases of a Pavlovian conditioning controlled experiment in which the UCS consisted of mental stress (counting backwards by 17s), the CS consisted of a 60-db buzzer 500 HZ), and the UCR cum CR was measured in terms of a decrement in ETCO2 from baseline. Positive evidence of conditioning of hyperventilation was found; the level of ETCO2 (CR) in response to the CS following four pairings of the CS and UCS was found to be significantly lower when compared with the level of ETCO2 in response to the CS prior to conditioning trials. Supplementary evidence of conditioning was found in corresponding measures of increased respiratory rate, increase heart rate, and increase electrodermal conductivity.

SUMMARY AND CONCLUSION

A reviews of a selection of research on respiration and the emotion of dyspnea/suffocation fear focused primary on panic disorder, the timely psychophysiological disorder that clearly illustrates the complex interaction between respiration and emotion in psychosomatic disease. In addition to the significant contribution made to the study of respiratory psychophysiology and related disorders, the research discussed here underscores the unifying paradigm provided by Pavlovian/classical conditioning. New directions in the study of dyspnea/suffocation fear in respiratory psychophysiology point to exploration of the parameters of conditioned hyperventilation and the search for clinical applications in diagnosis and treatment.

REFERENCES

(1) Ley R (1989) Dyspneic-fear and catastrophic cognitions in hyperventilatory panic attacks. Behevior Research and Therapy 27: 549-554.

(2) Ley R (1992) The many faces of Pan: Psychological and physiological differences among three types of panic attacks. Behaviour Research and Therapy 30: 347-357.

(3) Anderson B, Ley R (1998, September) Loss of voluntary control of respiration during a dyspnea/suffocation panic attack precipitated by relaxation. Paper presented at the annual meeting of the International Society for the Advancement of Respiratory Psychophysiology. Perpignan, France.

(4) Cohen A, Barlow D, Blanchard E(1985) The psychophysiology of relaxation associated panic attacks. Journal of Abnormal Psychology 94: 96-101.

(5) Lader M, Mathews A (1970) Physiological changes during spontaneous panic attacks. Journal of Psychosomatic Research 14: 377-382.

(6) Ley R (1999) The modification of breathing behavior: Pavlovian and operant control in emotion and cognition. Behavior Modification 23: 441-479.

(7) Margraf J, Ehlers A, Roth W (1987) panic attack associated with perceived hear rate acceleration: A case report. Behavior Therapy 18: 84-89.

(8) Sanderson W, Rapee R, Barlow D (1988) Panic induction via inhalation of 5.5% CO_2 enriched air: A single subject analysis of psychological and physiological effects. Behaviour Research and Therapy 26: 333-335.

(9) James W (1892) In: Allport G (eds) Psychology: the briefer course. New York, Harper and Row.

(10) Aitken R, Zeally A, Rosenthal S (1970) Some psychological and physiological considerations of breathlessness. In:Porter R (eds) Breathing: Hering Breuer Centenary Symposium. Churchill, London.

(11) Howell J, Campbell E (eds)(1966) Breathlessness: Proceedings of an international symposium held on 7 and 8 in 1965 under the auspices of the University of Manchester. Philadelphia, F,A. Davis Co.

(12) Mahler DA (eds)(1990) Dyspnea. Mount Kisco, New York, Futura Pub. Co. Inc.

(13) Papp L, Coplan J, Klein D, Woods S, Shear K, Barlow D, Gorman J (1998, September) Respiratory correlates of treatment outcome in panic disorder. Paper presented at the annual meeting of the International Society for the Advancement of Respiratory Psychophysiology, Perpignan, France.

(14) Klein D (1993) False suffocation alarm, spontaneous panic, and related condition: An integrative hypothesis. Archives of General Psychiatry 50: 306-316.

(15) Ley R (1998) Pulmonary function and dyspnea/suffocation-fear theory of panic. Journal of Behavior Therapy and Experimental Psychiatry 29: 1-11.

(16) Fowler W (1954) Breaking point of breathing holding. Journal of Applied Physiology 6: 536-545.

(17) Ley R (1996) Panic attacks: Klein's false suffocation alarm, Taylor and Rachman's data, and Ley's dyspnea-fear theory. Archives of General Psychiatry 53: 83.

(18) Ley R (1997) Ondine's Curse, false suffocation alarms, trait/state suffocation fear and dyspnea/suffocation fear in panic attacks. Archives of General Psychiatry 54: 677-678.

(19) Asmundson GJ, Stein MB (1994) A preliminary analysis of pulmonary function in panic disorder: Implications for the dyspnea-fear theory. Journal of Anxiety Disorder 8: 63-69.

(20) Broadhurst PL (1957) Emotionality and the Yerkes-Dodson law. Journal of Experimental Psychology 54: 345-352.

(21) Leukel F, Quinton E (1964) Carbon dioxide effects on acquisition and extinction of avoidance behavior. Journal of Comparative and Physiological Psychology 57: 267-270.

(22) Campbell D, Sanderson RE, Laverty SG (1964) Characteristics of a conditioned response in human subjects during extinction trials following a single traumatic conditioning trial. Journal of Abnormal and Social Psychology 68: 627-639.

(23) Mongeluzi D, Rosellini R, Caldarone B, Stock H, Abrahamsen G (1996) Pavlovian aversive context conditioning using carbon dioxide as the unconditioned stimulus. Journal of Experimental Psychology 22: 244-257.

(24) Mongeluzi D, Caldarone B, Stock H, Rosellini R, Ley R (Submitted) The conditioning of dyspneic fear in the white rat: Effectiveness of carbon dioxide at various concentrations and trace intervals.

(25) Dekker E, Pelser HE, Groen J (1957) Conditioning as a cause of asthma attacks. Journal of Psychosomatic Research 2: 97-108.

(26) Kotses H, Westlund R, Greer TL (1987) Performing mental arithmetic increases total respiratory resistance in individuals with normal respiration. Psychophysiology 24: 678-684.

(27) Miller D, Kotses H (1995) Classical conditioning of total respiratory resistance in humans. Psychosomatic Medicine 57: 148-153.

(28) Lum LC (1976) The syndrome of habitual chronic hyperventilation. In: Hill OW (eds) Modern Trend in Psychosomatic Medicine (Vol 3). London, Butterworth, pp196-230.

(29) Ley R, Ley J, Bassett C (1996) Pavlovian conditioning of hyperventilation. Supplement to Psychophysiology 33: 55.

Coordination of Breathing between Ribcage and Abdomen in Emotional Arousal

Hiroki Takase and Yutaka Haruki
School of Human Sciences, Waseda University, 2-579-15 Mikajima, Tokorozawa, Saitama 359-1192, JAPAN

Summary: This chapter discusses research of breathing patterns, especially coordination of the ribcage and the abdomen in conditions where a subject goes through a task that arouses in him/her negative or positive emotional states. The tasks that arouse negative emotional states were a mental arithmetic task and a reaction time task or to watch a videotaped scene. Two levels of materials were prepared for each of the tasks that were different in difficulty or stressfulness. In addition, the task which arouses positive emotional states was a muscle relaxation technique. These studies used as the measurement of the coordination, the relative phase between breathing movements of the ribcage and the abdomen. These results demonstrated that the fluctuations of the relative phase significantly increased from the pre-baseline period to the difficult or stressful task execution period. This showed that coordination of the ribcage and the abdomen deteriorated during stressful situations. On the other hand, the results of the experiment showed that coordination of the ribcage and the abdomen improved in a relaxed condition. The fluctuations that were found in these experiments, from the perspective of James' emotional theory, are discussed. These studies suggest that a perspective of dynamical systems is effective in studying emotion.

Keywords: Breathing, Coordination, Emotion, Task, Dynamical systems approach

William James, with his functionalistic view on emotion, argues that every animal behavior is effective in adapting itself to the environment. In James' approach, then, the physical responses that involve emotion are an animal's tendency to react to such specific conditions [1].

In Japanese, there are expressions such as "to be out of breath" or "to be breathless," "to catch one's breath," "to take one's breath away." These expressions not only literally describe human breathing activities, but also metaphorically express one's behavior and, in particular, mental/emotional states. The expressions are called "*karada kotoba* (literally 'body words')" and are used in everyday life. This suggests that, at least in Japan, the breathing activity is closely related to mental states. Under strained situations such as sporting events, musical recitals and public speech, we experience our breath rising, that is, our breathing becomes shallow and fast. On the other hand, when we are released from such a strained situation, tension reduces and as a result of relaxation, the breath that has been accumulated (i.e., heaped up) to that point is released. In other words, one regains a regular breathing pattern.

This chapter discusses investigation of breathing patterns in conditions where a subject goes through a task that arouses in him/her positive or negative emotional states. In so doing, a perspective in which the breathing movement is viewed as a dynamic organizing system while demonstrating its validity will be introduced.

I. Theoretical backgrounds of coordination

Task and Breathing

In research on the relationship between breathing and emotion, the breathing movements of the subjects are measured while they perform a mental arithmetic task and a reaction time task or watch a videotaped scene from a surgery or an car accident. To set up stressful conditions, instructions are given to the subject regarding an increase or decrease of a reward depending on his/her performance of the task, or regarding an electric shock that would be given to him/her as a punishment for failing to achieve a required level of performance. Consistent results obtained in such experiments are increases in respiration rate and in minute ventilation (reviewed in [2] [3]). Although limited in number, there are a few studies demonstrating that the post expiratory pause time may decrease under stressful conditions based on component analyses of every cycle of breathing movement [4] [5] [6].

Most of these results are obtained from observations of the amount of ventilation or the breathing movement of the ribcage. The breathing movement (ventilation) is mainly carried out by up-down movements of the diaphragm, and the expansion and contraction of the ribcage is caused by the contraction of intercostal muscles. In other words, breathing movements are achieved by movements of the abdominal muscles and those of the ribcage muscles. Grossman [7] suggests that both movements should be measured simultaneously since the ribcage and the abdomen may constrict independently from each other. Some, if not many, studies have already implemented Grossman's insight suggesting that the breathing amplitude of the ribcage either decreases or remains intact and that of the abdomen increases when positive emotion arises by watching a enjoyable film; in other words, the breathing pattern becomes abdominal dominant in such conditions [8] [9] [10]. In contrast, it is further suggested that when negative emotion is provoked in the subject by having him/her watch an unpleasant film or perform difficult tasks, the amplitude of the abdomen either decreases or remains intact and that of the ribcage increases; in other words, the breathing pattern becomes thoracic dominant in such conditions [8] [9] [10]. In summary, these studies demonstrate that the symmetric relationship between movement of the ribcage and that of the abdomen in breathing changes as a function of the kind of emotion that is being aroused.

Coordination

As previously mentioned, the breathing movement of human beings is mainly done by movement of the internal and external intercostal muscles and that of the diaphragm. Accordingly, the breathing movement can be observed as expansion and contraction of the ribcage and the abdomen. In order to carry out ventilation adequately, proper coordination between the movement of the ribcage and that of the abdomen is necessary. Coordination of the two movements is not static, but intrinsically dynamic, however, as should be clear from the fact that there are different breathing modes such as "thoracic breathing" and "abdominal breathing." Dynamic fluctuation, it seems, originates from the difference in inherent frequencies between the movement of the ribcage and that of the abdomen, which is, in turn, attributable to the differences in the structure, the muscle forces, the connections with the neural systems, etc. of the two different body parts.

A simple movement such as "walking" can not even be achieved by movements of the legs alone but which involves movements of many other body parts. The same goes with breathing which involves a large number of musculoskeletal and neural systems as sub-systems. In recent years, an increasing number of studies have approached the organization of body movements from the viewpoint that it is a self-organization of numerous sub-systems. The approach taken in these studies is called a "dynamical systems approach" and has brought new findings and insights into the studies of coordination among different body segments, of which intra-limb coordination among arms and legs is an example.

Pioneering research on the coordination phenomenon of an animal's body segments was conducted in the 1930's by Erich von Holst [11], a behavioral physiologist. Observing the movements of various kinds of animals, von Holst recognized the need to understand coordination as a function of temporary assemblages of multiple underlying subsystems. Von Holst's research on the coordination between the fins on both sides of a Labrus, a fish that swims with its longitudinal immobile axis, is an exemplary research case. The fins of a Labrus are independent from each other and oscillate at their own tempo. To achieve the behavior of "swimming," however, the fins must oscillate synchronously at a common tempo. Von Holt observed two tendencies. First, the oscillation of one of the fins tends to be attracted to that of the other fin, and this he calls the "magnet effect." Secondly, each of the fins tends not to abandon, but instead maintain its own inherent frequency when they start oscillating cooperatively. He called this the "maintenance tendency." It is emphasized that the maintenance tendency continues to remain even when the movements of the fins are perfectly coordinated to each other. That is to say that each fin maintains its own intrinsically dynamical nature while synchronizing itself with the oscillation of the other fin. The inter-fin coordination can be viewed, then, as a compromise between the cooperative mode or the magnetic effect, and the competitive mode or the maintenance tendency among the fins.

Coupled Oscillator Dynamics

Being largely influenced by von Holst's observation on physical coordination, a number of research studies have demonstrated that the behavior of the nervous and/or muscloskeltal systems in animals is a result of dynamical processes of self-organization. These studies can be characterized by their methodology called "dynamical systems approach" which have proposed models of formation and breakdown of stable patterns in intralimb coordination. Examples of such models include those of various rhythmic intra-/interlimb coordinations of a pair of limbs and multiple limbs (e.g., [12] [13]) within a single person on the one hand, and of multiple limbs across two people on the other (e.g., [14] [15]). The common thread that runs through all these studies is the identical principle of coordination which is at play in these various phenomena, thus pointing to the universal validity of these models of rhythmic coordination.

The studies on intralimb coordination have used as a measurement of coordination, the relative phase (ϕ) between two oscillating limbs. The ϕ indicates the "qualitative" spatio-temporal pattern of coordination between the rhythmic units. In the case of two limbs (e.g., the right and left arms) oscillating in the same tempo, ϕ is defined as the 0 radian if the two limbs are simultaneously at the same position in their cycle (referred to as "inphase mode"), and it is defined to be the π radian if simultaneously at the diametrically opposite position in the cycle (referred to as "antiphase mode"). Using the ϕ as a unit of analysis of intralimb coordination, research has focused on the question of whether and how the ϕ of intralimb changes when parameters apparently relevant to the behavior of intralimb coordination are manipulated (e.g., the frequency of oscillation of limbs).

Multiple areas of studies including physics, chemistry, biology, ecology, etc., have observed the phenomena of "self-organization" in which the macroscopic mode emerges from chaotic states to form a well-oraganized spatio-temporal structure. Most of these studies have been conducted in the field of "synergetics" [16]. In synergetics, the dependent variable, ϕ, is called an "order parameter" and describes the macroscopic structure of the system. The independent variables are called "control parameters," examples of which include the frequency of oscillation of the coupled intralimb system, ω_c, and the difference between the inherent frequencies of the underlying rhythmic unit (e.g., the left leg or the right leg in a walk), $\Delta\omega$. Using these parameters, studies have investigated the dynamics of order parameters between limbs in conditions where the control parameters were manipulated. The method used in synergetics enables us to mathematically model the behavior of the "order parameter," a "collective variable" that changes as a function of the "control parameter."

Based on these investigations, a model of the dynamics of the relative phase ϕ can be given as follows:

$$\dot{\phi} = \delta - a\sin(\phi) - 2b\sin(2\phi) + \sqrt{Q}\zeta \qquad (1)$$

Equation (1) is an order parameter equation, and $\dot{\phi}$ is the change rate of the relative phase. δ is equated to the difference between inherent frequencies (ω_i) of oscillators in question $\Delta\omega = (\omega_1 - \omega_2)$ (e.g., [12] [17] [18]). The ratio (b/a) of the coefficients a and b decides the strength of the coupling (coordination) between the oscillators. "$\sqrt{Q}\zeta$" is a stochastic noise process that arises from the multiplicity of the underlying subsystems [19]. Equation (1) predicts that the mean of the ϕ moves away from $\phi = 0$, π, and the standard deviation of ϕ increases, when the frequency of the oscillation increases. Equally, the equation predicts the same when the differences $\Delta\omega$ of the inherent frequency increase.

In the field of human physiology, research has begun from synergetics or dynamical systems perspectives (e.g., [20]).

Because breathing movements of the ribcage and the abdomen are periodic, each is considered as one oscillator. These two oscillators must construct one "breathing system" in order to make the air flow into or out of body by decreasing or increasing the pleural pressure. Therefore, how could we determine whether two oscillators are coordinative quantitatively ?

The dynamical systems approach proposes a method which uses the phase relation, especially the relative phase (or the mean of the relative phase, mean ϕ) and the standard deviation of the relative phase (SD ϕ). The ϕ (or mean ϕ) characterizes the coordinative relation between oscillators, and the SD ϕ, which expresses the variability of the ϕ, is an indicator of stability of coordination. For example, ϕ of both legs is about π radian, and the SD is restrained small by a usual walk. However, when weight is put on the leg, it will come to feel that it is difficult to move both legs alternately in a $\phi = \pi$ radian. At such time, the mean ϕ generally becomes the value apart from the π radian, and the SD ϕ becomes larger, and walking becomes "awkward." In general, the SD ϕ becomes larger around the transition from a stable movement state to another stable state (e.g., the transition from a "walk" to a "run") [21] [22] [23].

Up to the present, most studies on the breathing mode have tended to examine the amplitude independently and only show the differences between the ribcage and the abdomen. Few studies have investigated the phase relation between the ribcage and the abdomen quantitatively, however. The following is an introduction and discussion of new studies by the present author, which focus on the relative phase of movements of the ribcage and the abdomen (i.e., an index of coordination) both in stressful and relaxed situations. Let us first discuss the breathing patterns in a stressful setting.

II. Study I: Breathing pattern in the stressful condition

This study examined the breathing activities of participants when performing three different tasks of the same kind that have been commonly used in research to create a stressful situation. The tasks were an arithmetic task, a reaction time task and a stress film task.

Method
The participants were 12 undergraduate and graduate students at Waseda University (6 males and 6 females; the range of age in years was 19 to 23). The tasks were to perform a mental arithmetic task (henceforth, MA), a reaction time task (RT), and to watch a stressful film (FL). For each task, two levels of materials were prepared for each of the tasks differing in difficulty or stressfulness. Hence, we had as stimuli two difficult tasks (MA-D, RT-D) and one stressful film (FL-S), and two easy tasks (MA-E, RT-E) and one neutral film (FL-N). These tasks were presented to the participants in the order of easy/neutral tasks to difficult/stressful tasks. The content of the tasks were as follows:

In an MA task, the participant saw an incomplete equation presented on the computer display placed approximately 50 cm from him/her. For each question, he/she was instructed to click on the STOP button on the computer display with the mouse when he/she finished a calculation, immediately after which four multiple choice answers were displayed on the screen. The participant had to choose one answer from the choices that fit his/her own by clicking the mouse. For the difficult task (MA-D), additions of three-digit integers were used (e.g., 358 + 624 =), each of which had to be answered within four seconds. For the easy task (MA-E), additions of one-digit integers were used (e.g., 6 + 9 =) with no time limit in answering the questions. In both levels of tasks, a feedback sound was given each time the participant answered a question to let him/her know whether his/her answer was correct. In addition, the cumulative numbers of correct and incorrect answers were displayed on the computer monitor throughout the tasks to put pressure on the subjects.

In the RT task, the participant was asked to click with the mouse on the STOP button on the computer display when an asterisk was shown. For the difficult task (RT-D), the subject had to click the mouse as quickly as possible after the figure was presented. The performance was counted as correct when the participant succeeded in clicking the mouse within 0.350-seconds after the asterisk appeared. If the participant clicked on the mouse after more than 0.350 seconds or before the figure was presented, the performance was counted as an error. The interval of figure presentations was randomized within a range of 2 to 15 seconds. For the easy task (RT-E), the participants had to click the mouse when a figure appeared on the computer screen, but there was no time limit to achieve. The interval of figure presentation was fixed at 6 seconds. In RT-D only, a feedback sound was given to the subject after each performance to let him/her know the results. The cumulative numbers of correct answers and errors were indicated on the computer display throughout the tasks.

In the FL task, a videotaped scene of an ophthalmological surgery was presented as a stressful film (FL-S), and a videotaped psychological lecture on perception was used as a neutral film (FL-N).

The tasks MA, RT and FL were given in this order. The FL task had to be given at the end of the experiment to avoid strong and long-lasting influences observed in the preliminary experiment of the stressful film on the subjects' emotional states and, hence, on their performances of the other tasks. With this order, the subjects were predicted to get more used to the experimental situations as the experiment proceeded because of the repetitive nature of the tasks. Accordingly, the baseline data for 90 seconds were measured before each task was carried out.

The breathing movements were measured by Respiratory Inductive Plethysmograph (RIP, A. M. Inc.) attached to the circumference of the participant's ribcage (under the armpit) and of the abdomen (top of the navel).

Procedure. The participant was seated on a chair with the RIP attached to his/her ribcage and abdomen, with which the breathing data for a 5-minute baseline period were obtained. Following this, he/she carried out MA-E for 3 minutes and took a 3-minute rest as a post-baseline period. After 90 seconds of the pre-baseline period, the participant then carried out MA-D for 3 minutes. The exact same procedure was used for the RT and the FL tasks as well. For the difficult versions of the MA and RT tasks, participants were instructed that they would obtain more rewards after the experiment depending on the results of his/her task performances. That is, the more correct answers, the more rewards the participant earned.

Data analysis. Two methods of calculation of the relative phase were employed, The Peak method and the Valley method. In the Peak method the ϕ was calculated by using the time of maximum expansion of each breathing movement. In the Valley method the ϕ was calculated using the time of maximum contraction of each breathing movement (For more details see [24]).

Results

Respiration rate. In MA-E, MA-D and RT-D, the respiration rate significantly increased during the tasks from the pre-baseline and significantly decreased in the post-baseline period. These results were consistent for the breathing movements of the ribcage as well as those of the abdomen.

Mean ϕ and SD ϕ. Mean ϕ calculated by the Peak method significantly decreased from the pre-baseline period to the task execution period in MA-D. This result shows that the breathing pattern of the abdomen in the pre-baseline period was further strengthened during MA-D. Moreover, the SD ϕ significantly increased from the pre-baseline period to the task execution period and decreased significantly in the post-baseline period (Fig. 1). This shows that coordination of the ribcage and the abdomen deteriorated when carrying out difficult tasks. The mean ϕ obtained by the Valley method did not change significantly for any of the stressful tasks, namely MA-D, RT-D and FL-S. Moreover, the SD ϕ obtained by the same method significantly increased from the pre-baseline period to the task period and significantly decreased in the post-baseline. This demonstrates that coordination of the ribcage and the abdomen deteriorated during difficult or stressful tasks.

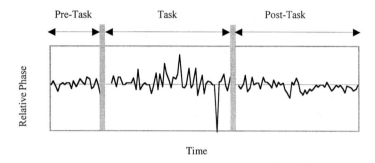

Fig.1. Time series of relative phase between breathing
movements of the ribcage and the abdomen

III. Study II: Breathing pattern in the relaxed condition

This study examined the breathing activities of the participants when they performed a relaxation technique.

Method

The participants were 28 undergraduate students at Waseda University (14 males and 14 females; the range of age in years was 18 to 23). A relaxation technique combining part of a simplified version of Jacobson's muscle relaxation and relaxation technique of the shoulder was used. The measurement of breathing movements and the data analysis were as the aforementioned experiment.

Procedure. The participant was seated on a chair with the RIP attached to his/her ribcage and abdomen, with which the breathing data for a 5-minute baseline period were obtained. Following this, he/she practiced the relaxation technique adequately. After mastering the technique, the participant performed the technique at his/her own pace and took a 3-minute rest as a post-baseline period.

Results

Respiration rate. The respiration rate significantly decreased from the pre-baseline period to the post-baseline period. These results were consistent for the breathing movements of the ribcage as well as those of the abdomen.

Mean ϕ and SD ϕ. The mean ϕ calculated by the Peak method significantly increased from the pre-baseline period to the post-baseline period. This result shows that the breathing pattern of the abdomen in the pre-baseline period was further strengthened in the post-baseline period. Moreover, the SD ϕ significantly decreased from the pre-baseline period to the post-baseline period. This shows that coordination of the ribcage and the abdomen improved after performing the technique. No significant changes were found in the mean ϕ and the SD ϕ calculated by the Valley method.

IV. General Discussion

Self-organizing Breathing Movements and James' Functionalism Theory

An increase in the SD ϕ between two oscillators indicates that coordination of the two oscillators has deteriorated. The experiment investigating breathing patterns in stressful conditions demonstrated that coordination of the breathing movements of the ribcage and the abdomen declined under stressful conditions (MA-D, RT-D, FL-S), because the SD ϕ (calculated by the Peak or the Valley method) increased.

The two movements oscillating in a coordinative mode under certain conditions disappear due to external or internal changes, and then construct a new coordinative mode again. This is the phenomenon seen every day, for example, as already stated, in a transition from a "walk" to a "run." From walking to running, the coordination between the left and the right legs specific to "walk" collapses and is taken over by the coordination specific to "run."

Kelso's [25] original research models the phenomenon of intralimb coordination. Kelso asked participants to oscillate their two index fingers at coupled frequency ω_c, specified by the metronome. When the coupled frequency ω_c increased gradually, the antiphase mode ($\phi = \pi$) of the index fingers switched abruptly to an inphase mode ($\phi = 0$) at a certain critical value. This is called "phase transition." This phase transition never occurs when two index fingers oscillate in antiphase mode with ω_c decreasing (the speed of oscillation slows down), or when two index fingers oscillate in an inphase mode initially with ω_c increasing. The SD ϕ is raised rapidly around this critical value. This shows that coordination collapses when a coordinative movement switches to another coordinative movement.

As stated at the beginning, William James thought that animal behavior is affected by adaptations to environment [1]. From James' viewpoint, weakening of the coordination of the ribcage and the abdomen following stressful conditions (MA-D, RT-D, FL-S) is defined as the exploratory process in which breathing movements of the ribcage and the abdomen oscillating cooperatively during pre-baseline collapse and construct a new coordination to adapt to the novel environment. At this time, if the intensity of the stressful condition is relatively weak, a new coordinative relation between the ribcage and the abdomen suitable for the situation is immediately formed (the "magnet effect" becomes predominant over the "maintenance tendency" which von Holst defined). If the stress intensity is strong, it is not easy to reconstruct breathing coordination. If the intensity of stress is too strong, the coordinative movements of the ribcage and the abdomen may continue to disappear with the unusual or abnormal breathing possibly causing paradoxical breathing in which the "maintenance tendency" is larger. On the contrary, under a relaxed condition, breathing pattern seems to change quickly to a stable coordinative behavior as revealed by the experimental results in this chapter.

Asymmetry of Inspiration and Expiration

The breathing pattern in the FL-S task, the decline of the coordination did increase in the SD ϕ used by the Valley method, but the similar result was not found in the Peak method. In the results in the relaxed condition the same results were found by using the two methods. These results used by two methods indicated that which reference points would be selected in the techniques in order to get the results. It can be speculated that this differences might be due to the qualitative differences between the ϕ at the points of maximum expansion (used in the Peak method) and that at the points of maximum contraction (used in the Valley method).

The ϕ calculated by the Peak method are the lags of the end points of inspiration or the start points of expiration between the ribcage and the abdomen, and the ϕ calculated by the Valley method are the lags of the end points of expiration or the start points of inspiration between the ribcage and the abdomen. In large part, expiration progresses passively due to relaxation of the inspiratory muscle. In addition, it has been demonstrated that the post expiratory pause time decreases under stressful conditions. (The same results were found in the experimental data in this chapter as well though it isn't described in this chapter). From these results, it can be said that the post expiratory pause period is very sensitive to stressful situation as compared with the post inspiratory pause period. Consequently, it could be thought that the differences between the ϕ at the points of maximum expansion and that at the points of maximum contraction may arise from the fact that the circumference of maximum contraction is sensitive and especially instable in a stressful situation, and thus, the variability of the ϕ at the points of maximum contraction might be greater than that at the points of maximum expansion.

Validity of the perspective of dynamical systems theory in emotion research

Recently, dynamical systems approach research examining breathing movements of the ribcage and the abdomen of a preterm and a normal infant at the age of 38 post consepUonal showed that a preterm infant's coordination of breathing movements of the ribcage and the abdomen was less stable, and that the ϕ of the ribcage and the abdomen was larger than those of a normal infant [26]. Furthermore, it was possible to identify the preterm or the normal infant by ϕ of breathing movements of the ribcage and the abdomen, as well as predict the neurobehavioral examination score. The instability of coordination of a preterm infant results from the underdevelopment of the neural systems or musculoskeletal systems. However, similar phenomena have been observed in normal adults. It can be said that coordination of breathing movements of the ribcage and the abdomen is influenced by stressful tasks or relaxing-specific kinematic context.

Breathing movements of the ribcage and the abdomen are restricted by their own dynamical properties, such as mass or construction. For example, one study has showed that as the speed of breathing increases, the coordination of breathing movement of the ribcage and the abdomen lessens [27]. This could be explained by the fact that the difference in inherent frequencies of breathing movements of the ribcage and the abdomen increase the difference of movement cycle.

It is said that sympathetic nervous activity becomes predominant and muscles become tense when one experiences negative emotions, such as anxiety or tension. At this time, it seems that the physical properties of the breathing muscles of the ribcage and the abdomen grow *stiff*, and the dynamic properties and the dynamics change. As a result, the breathing movement becomes smaller and faster in general. At the same time, a difference between the tension of muscles of the ribcage and the abdomen is produced which causes the difference of inherent frequencies between the muscles to increase. There is an experimental paradigm of the "wrist-pendulum system" based on the dynamical systems theory for studying intralimb coordination [28]. In this paradigm, one holds two pendulums in one's hands and swings each pendulum about an axis in the wrist (with other joints fixed) parallel to the sagittal plane. This paradigm causes manipulation of the inherent frequency by changing the mass and the length of the pendulums. Many studies have demonstrated that the variability of ϕ between two pendulums increases when the difference in inherent frequencies of the hand-held pendulums is kept away from 0 (e.g., [13]). The equation of order parameter (1) predicts that the variability of ϕ increases, that is, the coordination between two oscillators is lower (weaker) when the coupled frequency of two oscillators or the difference of inherent frequencies between two oscillators increases.

V. Conclusion

William James emphasized that a "body" or a "physical changes" plays an important role in the formation and experience of emotion [29]. A body consists of various systems (e.g., central nervous system, circulation system, musculoskeletal system, etc.), which interact cooperatively [20]. This paper shows that coordination of the breathing movements of the ribcage and the abdomen which are subsystems of ventilation change dynamically when emotions are aroused. In emotion research, the dynamical systems theory is an effective methodology that approaches from the perspective of investigating the mutual relationship of subsystems underlying the body, and especially from the perspective of the coordination between the subsystems.

REFERENCES

1. Cornelius RR (1996) The Science of Emotion. Prentice-Hall, Inc.
2. Boiten F, Frijda NH, Wientjes JC (1994) Emotions and respiratory patterns: Review and critical analysis. International Journal of Psychophysiology 17:103-128
3. Grossman P (1983) Respiration, stress and cardiovascular function. Psychophysiology 20:284-300
4. Boiten FA (1993) Component analysis of task-related respiratory patterns. International

Journal of Psychophysiology 15:91-104

5. Cohen HD, Goodenough DR, Witkin HA, Oltman P, Gould H, Shulman E (1975) The effects of stress on components of the respiration cycle. Psychophysiology 12:377-380

6. Umezawa A (1991) Changes of respiratory activity during laboratory stress. Japanese Journal of Physiology Psychology and Psychophysiology 9:43-55 (Sutoresushigeki ni taisuru kokyuukatudou no henyou. Seirisinrigaku to seisinseirigaku)

7. Grossman SP (1967) A textbook of physiological psychology. Wiley, New York

8. Ancoli S, Kamiya J (1979) Respiratory patterns during emotional expression. Biofeedback Self-regulation 4:242

9. Ancoli S, Kamiya J, Ekman P (1980) Psychophysiological differentiation of positive and negative affects. Biofeedback Self-regulation 5:356-357

10. Svebak S (1975) Respiratory patterns as predictors of laughter. Psychophysiology, 12:62-65

11. von Holst E (1973) Relative coordination as a phenomenon and as a method of analysis of central nervous system function. In Martin R (ed & trans) The collected papers of Erich von Holst: Vol.1. The behavioral physiology of animal and man. University of Miami Press, pp 33-135 (Original work published 1939)

12. Kelso JAS, Jeka JJ (1992) Symmetry breaking dynamics of human multilimb coordination. Journal of Experimental Psychology: Human Perception and Performance 18:645-668

13. Schmidt RC, Shaw BK, Turvey MT (1993) Coupling dynamics in interlimb coordination. Journal of Experimental Psychology: Human Perception and Performance 19:397-415

14. Schmidt RC, Carello C, Turvey MT (1990) Phase transitions and critical fluctuations in the visual coordination of rhythmic movements between people. Journal of Experimental Psychology: Human Perception and Performance 16:227-247

15. Schmidt RC, Turvey MT (1994) Phase-entrainment dynamics of visually coupled rhythmic movements. Biological Cybernetics 70:369-376

16. Haken H (1978) Synergetics: An Introduction. Springer-Verlag, Berlin

17. Kelso JAS, DelColle JD, Schöner G (1990) Action-perception as a pattern formation process. In Jeannerod M (ed) Attention and performance XIII. Erlbaum, Hillsdale, NJ, pp 139-169

18. Rand R, Cohen AH, Holmes PJ (1988) Systems of coupled oscillators as models of central pattern generators. In Cohen AH, Rossignol S, Grillner S (eds) Neural control of rhythmic movements in verterbrates. (pp 333-367) Wiley, New York, pp 333-367

19. Schöner G, Haken H, Kelso JAS (1986) A stochastic theory of phase transitions in human hand movement. Biological Cybernetics 73:27-35

20. Haken H, Koepchen HP (eds) (1991) Rhythms in Physiological Systems. Springer-Verlag, Berlin

21. Kelso JAS (1995) Dynamic patterns: The self-organization of brain and behavior. MIT press, Cambridge

22. Kelso JAS, Scholz JP, Schöner G (1986) Nonequilibrium phase transitions in coordinated biological motion: Critical fluctuations. Physics Letters A 118:279-284

23. Turvey MT (1990) Coordination. American Psychologist 45:938-953

24. Yamanishi J, Kawato M, Suzuki R (1979) Studies on human finger tapping neural networks by phase transition curves. Biological Cybernetics 33:199-208

25. Kelso JAS (1984) Phase transitions and critical behavior in human bimanual coordination.

American Journal of Physiology: Regulatory, Integrative, and Comparative 246:R1000-R1004

26. Goldfield EC, Schmidt RC, Fitzpatrick P (1999) Coordination dynamics of abdomen and chest during infant breathing: A comparison of full-term and preterm infants at 38 weeks postconceptional age. Ecological Psychology 11:209-232

27. Schmidt RC (1997) Personal communication (Date: Mon, 22nd Sep.)

28. Kugler PN, Turvey MT (1987) Information, natural law and the self-assembly of rhythmic movement. Erlbaum, Hillsdale, NJ

29. James W (1884) What is an emotion? Mind 19:188-205

Behavioural and Physiological Factors Affecting Breathing Pattern and Ventilatory Control in Patients with Idiopathic Hyperventilation

Sandy Jack[1], MSc, Clinical Scientist
Mark Wilkinson[2], BSc (HONS), MBChB, MRCP, Clinical Research Fellow
Christopher J. Warburton[1, 2], MBChB, MD, MRCP, AFOM, Consultant Respiratory Physician

[1] Aintree Chest Centre, University Hospital Aintree, Lower Lane, Liverpool, L9 7AL, U.K.
[2] University Of Liverpool Dept of Medicine, Duncan Building, Liverpool, L69 3GA, UK.

Summary: Idiopathic Hyperventilation may be defined as breathing in excess of metabolic requirements, resulting in hypocapnia and concomitant respiratory alkalosis which is not associated with other cardio-respiratory disease. It is characterised both by an inappropriate level of ventilation and by a disorganised breathing pattern. Common symptoms reported by patients include shortness of breath, dizziness, chest tightness and parasthesia. High levels of anxiety have also been observed. The aetiology of this condition is unknown but is likely to be a combination of multiple factors, both psychological and physiological. Mechanical, chemical and behavioural elements are likely to be involved in the symptomatology. In this chapter, we discuss the history of idiopathic hyperventilation and explain how the diagnosis can be made. We demonstrate the variability of breathing pattern and suggest the mechanisms that may be involved in its maintenance. We also describe an index which may be useful in assessing and assigning a numerical value to this disorganised breathing pattern, which may prove to be useful for diagnostic purposes, for assessing progression or the effects of therapy. In addition we describe respiratory physiological changes observed in our laboratory in these subjects including an exaggerated ventilatory response both to low levels of exercise and to CO_2 when replaced to normocapnic levels. We demonstrate that these patients have a lower control point for CO_2 compared to normals and discuss how this altered chemoresponsiveness may partially explain the poor exercise tolerance and symptomatology in these individuals. We provide evidence that control point may be altered by behaviour which suggests that psychological factors may alter physiology in these individuals.

Key words: Hyperventilation, Behaviour, Breathing pattern, Ventilatory Control

INTRODUCTION

Idiopathic hyperventilation is an uncommon condition which causes a plethora of symptoms, causing patients to present to a wide variety of specialities. Idiopathic (or primary) hyperventilation is defined for the purposes of this chapter, as breathing in excess of metabolic requirements for which there is no demonstrable cardio-respiratory cause. The principle symptomatology of such patients involves respiratory symptoms and in particular shortness of breath and chest tightness are common. A typical presentation to the Chest Clinic is exercise limitation due to breathlessness, which is disproportionate to the level of lung function. Other symptoms such as parasthesia and dizziness are also relatively common. Hyperventilation is known also to occur in conjunction with many other conditions such as asthma, chronic obstructive pulmonary disease, ischaemic heart disease and causes of pain. Such secondary hyperventilation will not be dealt with in any detail in this chapter, although undoubtedly it does contribute significantly to the symptoms produced by the underlying co-morbidities.

HISTORICAL BACKGROUND

Symptoms consistent with idiopathic hyperventilation were described as far back as the 19th century. DaCosta [1] reported symptoms similar to idiopathic hyperventilation in soldiers in the American Civil war in 1871. These symptoms were thought at the time to be cardiac in origin, as the soldiers complained of chest tightness and shortness of breath (the syndrome being named *The Soldier's Irritable Heart* or *DaCosta's Syndrome*). It was not until 1908 that Haldane and Poulton [2] first described the effects of overbreathing. They suggested that the symptoms of painful tingling in the hands and feet with reduced cerebral blood flow may be due to changes in pH rather than $PaCO_2$. Collip and Backus [3] in 1920 proposed a link between hypocapnia and symptomatology, when they described that overbreathing could cause a reduction in arterial carbon dioxide levels of 44%. This was noted to be associated with the production of symptoms in their subjects. It was not until 1929 however that White and Hahn [4] suggested that *DaCosta's Syndrome* was actually caused by overbreathing and also noted the association with the symptoms of sighing and dyspnoea. Thompson [5] clarified the relationship between apparent cardiac abnormalities and DaCosta's Syndrome in 1943. He reported that overbreathing could cause electrocardiographic changes, which were thought largely to be related to the alkalosis produced by overbreathing.

The first description of a relationship between symptomatology consistent with idiopathic hyperventilation and psychological factors was published by Soley and Shock [6] in 1938, however it was not until Lowry's work in 1967 [7] that this was studied again. Lowry investigated the psychological aspects of idiopathic hyperventilation and suggested that it was identical to hysteria and that these patients considered themselves to be physically inferior and to have perfectionist's traits. More recently in 1976 Lum [8] has described the association between hyperventilation and psychology. Lum has proposed a theory that when hyperventilation and concomitant hypocapnia are triggered by anxiety, this creates symptoms which are perceived and interpreted by the patient. A vicious circle is then created whereby the symptoms are interpreted by the patient as the sensations experienced during life threatening illness, this creates further anxiety which worsens the hyperventilation and symptoms.

Ley [9] has also proposed a theory linking hyperventilation with psychology, this time the clinical entity of panic attacks. The primary symptoms reported during panic attacks are dyspnoea and tachycardia, which may be as a consequence of hyperventilatory hypocapnia and the mechanical effort of overbreathing. Panic and fear may occur as a result of dyspnoea and subsequent catastrophic thought may be due to cerebral hypoxia caused by cerebral vasoconstriction due to hypocapnia. The relationship between idiopathic hyperventilation and panic attacks is however unclear. Undoubtedly panic attacks are frequently associated with hyperventilation during the attack, however we feel that there is limited overlap between the two conditions. Patients with panic attacks have easily definable "attacks" associated with fear, whereas patients with true idiopathic hyperventilation do not experience fear but develop symptoms attributable to their overbreathing. In these patients the conditioned response to stress (either physical in the form of exercise, or psychological such as anxiety) appears abnormal and as a result of this they overbreathe. These episodes of hyperventilation in response to stress however generally do not cause panic or fear in the patient. A more accurate definition of the two patient groups may be to describe them as *"panic attack patients"* who will experience symptoms related to acute hyperventilation during an attack alone and *"chronic idiopathic hyperventilators"* who experience symptoms from their more chronic hyperventilation each day of their life both at rest and on exercise.

DISEASE MECHANISMS AND DIAGNOSIS

Both mechanical and chemical factors may contribute to the vast range of symptomatology experienced by patients with idiopathic hyperventilation. In addition psychological factors may also play a role. Dizziness and parasthesia may be related to hypocapnia, as this is known to cause peripheral, cerebral and coronary vasoconstriction. The mechanical effort of overbreathing is thought to contribute to sensations of dyspnoea and chest tightness and therefore abolition of hypocapnia during hyperventilation may not abolish all of the symptoms associated with hyperventilation.

Diagnosis of idiopathic hyperventilation involves the demonstration of hyperventilation in the absence of significant cardio-respiratory disease. Various forms of provocation tests have been described including voluntary overbreathing (which is still thought by some to be the "gold standard"), mental stress challenge and exercise testing. The demonstration of reduced end-tidal carbon dioxide levels is the usual criterion for diagnosis. A level of less than 32 mmHg which is sustained, for at least a minute at rest or on exercise is a useful cut-off level for normality. Variability in minute ventilation is also seen in some patients with idiopathic hyperventilation during rest, early exercise and recovery from exercise and may also suggest the underlying diagnosis. This will be discussed in more detail later in this chapter.

Voluntary overbreathing (also often termed a hyperventilation provocation test) causes significant symptoms in both normal individuals and patients with idiopathic hyperventilation. A recent study by Hornsveld [10] has suggested that the test itself is not useful for diagnostic purposes for this very reason. We feel however that although it is true that the symptoms produced do not differentiate normality from idiopathic hyperventilation, the behaviour of subjects after the voluntary overbreathing stops can be very instructive. In normal subjects as a result of hypocapnia, minute ventilation is rapidly reduced to pre-test levels (or below), whereas patients with idiopathic hyperventilation continue to overbreathe with sustained hypocapnia for at least several minutes.

In addition to the delayed time to recovery following hyperventilation provocation testing, reduced breath hold time is also a consistent feature in patients with idiopathic hyperventilation. This mean breath hold time is around 25% of the time demonstrated by normal subjects and is not improved by performing the breath hold using 100% oxygen (which in normals will increase breath hold time by 50%). The Buteyko method of treatment for asthma involves training in breath hold and it is possible that part of the symptomatic benefit demonstrated by this treatment may in fact be related to improvement of underlying hyperventilation (which has been demonstrated to occur in a significant number of asthmatics).

Data from our laboratory would suggest that cardio-respiratory exercise testing is the most reliable method of diagnosing idiopathic hyperventilation. This is our "gold-standard" for diagnosis. Patients demonstrate a characteristic pattern of exercise response with inappropriately high minute ventilation during exercise, reduced end-tidal carbon dioxide tensions and a disorganised breathing pattern. Their exercise capacity is reduced however there is usually little evidence of ventilatory or cardiac limitation. The mechanism of exercise limitation in such patients is unclear but may relate to poor motivation, respiratory or leg muscle fatigue or may be due to an effect on exercising muscle of the alkalosis produced by hyperventilation. The large rise in ventilation at peak exercise (respiratory compensation) is seldom witnessed in idiopathic hyperventilators and may be due to the lactic acidosis being offset by the pre-existing alkalosis. The arterial blood pH in this situation seldom falls below normal and therefore does not stimulate respiratory compensation.

We have demonstrated in our laboratory that this inappropriate ventilatory response to exercise is further exaggerated when the end-tidal carbon dioxide is artificially maintained within the physiological range. Exercise tolerance during carbon dioxide replacement is not improved and symptoms are not wholly abolished (in fact chest tightness and breathlessness are worsened).

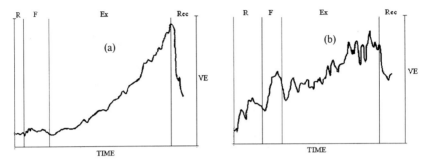

Fig.1 Ventilation (L/min) during rest (R), freewheel (F), incremental exercise (E) and recovery (Rec) in a normal subject (a) and a subject with idiopathic hyperventilation (b).

Patients with idiopathic hyperventilation report a wide variety of symptoms. For diagnostic purposes these symptoms may be assessed using the Nijmegen questionnaire [11]. This questionnaire was designed as an aid to diagnosis and was found to adequately separate hyperventilators from non-hyperventilators (a score of 23 out of 64 indicating hyperventilation). It also appears useful as a quantifying instrument for evaluating the effects of therapeutic intervention in these patients [12].

MECHANISMS OF VENTILATORY STABILITY

During exercise, patients with idiopathic hyperventilation demonstrate a disorganised breathing pattern, which is unrelated to metabolic demands [13]. It has previously been demonstrated that hyperventilation, the concomitant hypocapnia and respiratory alkalosis may be related to stress and anxiety. It is possible that increased anxiety and other psychological factors may alter homeostatic mechanisms, although the exact mechanism by which this is achieved is not clear. Plum [14] proposed a model of interaction of emotional disturbance and the motor behavioural pathway. The motor behavioural pathway functions in addition to the metabolic pathway of ventilatory control. It is thought that copies of motor signals from respiratory muscles (corollary discharge) are sent to areas of the cortex where they are perceived as sensations of effort. Patients with idiopathic hyperventilation may have an inappropriate perception of work, which makes them feel that their exertion is extreme and they require to ventilate at high level. This feeling self-perpetuates. Recent data suggests that higher neural centre stimulus may affect breathing pattern by altering breathing frequency. It has also been shown using the Dipole tracing method that these higher neural centres are stimulated during anticipatory anxiety [15]. This evidence would suggest that psychological factors may have a profound effect on respiratory control mechanisms.

The inappropriate breathing pattern observed during exercise may be due to a variety of factors. Hypocapnia alone is known to cause unstable breathing patterns [16]. At times of low metabolic activity, behavioural mechanisms may override physiological mechanisms and have potentially their greatest effect [17]. We have observed anecdotally that patients with idiopathic hyperventilation demonstrate greater variability in breathing pattern during low to moderate work rates, however this variability becomes more normal as work rate increases towards anaerobic threshold and peak. This would suggest that the breathing pattern might be governed by behavioural factors when metabolic demand is low and becomes driven by metabolic requirements at higher work rates.

Instability of ventilation may be due to a variety of other factors. There may be increased peripheral relative to central chemosensitivity to carbon dioxide [18] as well as uncoordinated upper airways and chest wall muscles. Patients with idiopathic hyperventilation are known to a have a thoracic pattern of breathing which may contribute to this inappropriate breathing pattern. As a result of the interaction between chemical (metabolic) and non-chemical (behavioural) drives at rest and during early exercise there may be random variations in ventilation from breath to breath. In fully established hyperventilation this apparent instability of the ventilatory control system may become a conditioned response to stress or exercise and is perpetuated.

Quantification of the variability in breathing pattern has rarely been studied in patients with idiopathic hyperventilation. To evaluate this non-metabolic response to exercise, we assessed the breathing pattern in early exercise of normal patients and idiopathic hyperventilators. The latter are defined for the purposes of this study, as experiencing an end-tidal carbon dioxide level of less than 30mmHg for more than 1 minute during exercise. Patients performed a maximal symptom limited cardio-respiratory exercise test on a cycle ergometer. Measurements were recorded on a computerised breath by breath exercise system. Patients exercised to volitional termination using a ramped protocol of 15 or 20 watts per minute of exercise depending on physical fitness. Breath by breath ventilatory equivalent for oxygen (VE/VO_2) was analysed during the first half of exercise. This methodology was used to ensure subjects remained below anaerobic threshold and to ensure a linear response of VE/VO_2 to exercise. We excluded the first 30 seconds of pedalling to allow breathing pattern to stabilise at the onset of exercise.

The VE/VO_2 is derived from ventilatory parameters and may be used as a measure of the appropriateness of ventilation. A high level of the ratio would suggest that a large breath (VE) was taken in the absence of a significant oxygen requirement (VO_2). In contrast, a low value of this ratio would suggest relative hypoventilation in response to a significant oxygen requirement. The normal range for VE/VO_2 is 20-28.

We studied 20 patients with idiopathic hyperventilation, 7 males, 13 females with a mean age (SD) of 53(11) years. In addition 18 normal patients, 9 males, 9 females with a mean age (SD) of 47(12) years were studied for comparison. The group mean VE/VO_2 was 27 (range 21 – 31) for normal patients during the first half of exercise with a standard deviation (SD) of 1.8 (range 1.1 – 4). This compared to a group mean $VE/VO2$ of 55 (range 28-93) with SD 12 (range 4-28) in patients with idiopathic hyperventilation. Neither the mean nor the SD alone adequately separated the groups, although the SD was close to achieving this aim. Both mean $VE/VO2$ and the standard deviation of VE/VO_2 were greater in the hyperventilation group but there was overlap between the two groups. As a discriminator therefore both the level and variability of VE/VO_2 would appear important and therefore we derived an index to take into account both these factors. The Exercise Breathing Index (EBI) was derived as the mean multiplied by the standard deviation of VE/VO_2 during the first half of exercise for each subject. The group mean EBI for normal patients was 49 with a range of 27 to 112. For the patients with idiopathic hyperventilation the mean EBI was 693 with a range of 120 to 1900.

This index was shown therefore to adequately separate normals from idiopathic hyperventilators, although some normal subjects had relatively high levels of EBI. These subjects would appear to have some instability in their breathing pattern without evidence of hypocapnia. The significance of this is unclear and the symptomatology of these patients needs to be studied to ascertain whether they are mild (or recent onset) hyperventilators. We found no correlation of EBI with end-tidal CO_2 levels in the idiopathic hyperventilators ($r = -0.33$ $p = NS$) and we believe that this index may be a useful way of quantifying the severity of idiopathic hyperventilation which is more sensitive than only using end-tidal CO_2 levels. At the very least the EBI is a way of documenting and assigning a numeric value to the disorganised and inappropriate breathing pattern of patients with idiopathic hyperventilation.

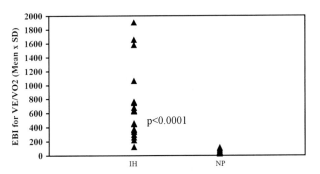

Fig 2.   EBI For VE/VO2 on Normal Patients (NP) and Idiopathic Hyperventilators (IH)

We have since tested different groups of normals and patients with idiopathic hyperventilation and again found that the EBI adequately separates normality from hyperventilators.

To assess the effect on the EBI of normalising CO_2 levels during exercise in hyperventilators we have studied 15 patients with idiopathic hyperventilation (11 females, 4 males - mean age (SD) 54.8 (12) years during hypocapnic and normocapnic exercise. Patients performed two symptom limited cardio-respiratory exercise tests as previously described. During one exercise test end-tidal CO_2 was maintained within the physiological range of 40 to 42 mmHg. This was achieved by titrating 100% CO_2 into the inspired limb of a biased flow circuit incorporating a partial rebreathe. We measured the change in breathing pattern parameters, including the EBI and the ratio of time of inspiration to total respiratory cycle time (Ti/Ttot), a measure of respiratory timing under both these conditions. There was no significant change in the EBI on CO_2 replacement during the first half of exercise. There was however a reduction in the Ti/Ttot ratio on normocapnic exercise suggesting a reduction in inspiratory time during normocapnia. The change in Ti/Ttot from hypocapnic to normocapnic exercise was compared to anxiety scores derived from the Hospital Anxiety and Depression scores (HADs) for each subject and showed a significant negative correlation ($r = 0.51$ $p<0.05$).

This would suggest that the more severe the anxiety level in an individual, the more of an effect CO_2 replacement had on the ventilatory response to exercise. This in turn would suggest that the higher the level of anxiety, the higher and more abnormal the ventilatory response is in patients with idiopathic hyperventilation during mild to moderate levels of exercise during CO_2 replacement.

It is known that psychological factors, in particular chronic anxiety, are associated with irregularities of breathing pattern In particular this is mediated by increases in respiratory rate without a metabolic stimulus. Ventilatory inefficiency as reflected by an increase in VE/VO2 ratio has also been observed in high-trait-anxiety groups.

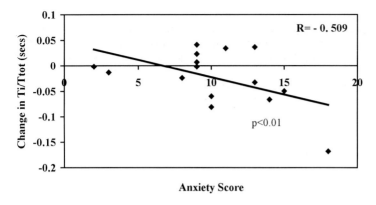

Fig 3. Correlation of Change in Ti/Ttot between Hypocapnic and Normocapnic Exercise with Anxiety

To investigate the influence of behavioural factors and normocapnia on breathing pattern at low to moderate work rates compared to higher work rates we studied a different group of 8 patients with idiopathic hyperventilation (4 males, 4 females, mean age (SD) 59(4) years) during hypocapnic and normocapnic exercise tests. Breathing pattern was once again assessed during the first 60 watts of exercise from 30-second averaged intervals using mean and SD for VE/VO_2. The results are tabulated below in Table 1.

Table 1. Comparison of VE/VO_2 During Hypocapnic and Normocapnic Exercise Tests

EXERCISE			EXERCISE + CO2		
Watts	Mean	SD	Watts	Mean	SD
0	49.6(13)	12.9 (6)	0	56.1(14)	13.5(6)
8	44.9(17)[#]	7.9 (7)	9	59.6(10)[#]	6.9 (6)*
17	47.3(17)[#]	10.9(8)[#]	17	60.2(10)[#]	3.7 (3)*[#]
23	47.3(15)[#]	6.2 (3)*	25	60.7(10)[#]	3.8 (2)*
61	43.5(13)	4.9 (4)*[#]	63	54.3 (9)	3.2 (2)*[#]

* $p<0.05$ value different from rest value
\# $p<0.05$ value for comparison of exercise to exercise + CO_2

Mean VE/VO_2 did not alter significantly on either exercise test from respective resting levels. The mean VE/VO_2 was higher during normocapnic exercise than during hypocapnic exercise demonstrating an augmented ventilatory response to normocapnia. This will be discussed in more detail below.

The variability of VE/VO_2 as measured by the standard deviation was significantly higher at resting levels and during early exercise compared to higher work rates on both hypocapnic and normocapnic exercise tests. The decreased variability in breathing pattern at higher metabolic demands during the hypocapnic exercise test would suggest that at lower work rates behavioural factors do indeed predominate and at the higher levels variability reduces significantly towards more normal levels. This change is driven probably by metabolic factors. During normocapnic exercise there was also less variability in VE/VO_2 compared to the hypocapnic test at all work rates, significant at the 5% level at a work rate of 17 watts. Variability appeared to decrease earlier and to a greater level during normocapnic exercise. This would suggest that hypocapnia may in fact contribute to instability of ventilation. This result surprised us, as the results in the previous section had not shown a change in EBI during normocapnic exercise at low work rates. This apparent conflicting data can be rationalised if one considers the statistical composition of the EBI. With CO_2 replacement during exercise the mean VE/VO_2 increases whilst the SD of VE/VO_2 decreases. By multiplying these two values together to derive the EBI the effect of increasing one is offset by the reduction in the other thus the EBI may not change significantly and will be dependant upon the relative magnitude of the increases and decreases involved. The rise in ventilation as a result of CO_2 replacement suggested to us that there may be an increased sensitivity to CO_2 in patients with idiopathic hyperventilation with increased levels of inappropriate ventilation.

The effect of abolishing hypocapnia on breathing pattern was further investigated by analysing EBI at intervals during exercise from rest to 60 watts during hypocapnic and normocapnic exercise. These results are presented in Table 2.

Table 2. EBI During Hypocapnic and Normocapnic Exercise Tests

Watts	EBI	Watts	EBI
	EXERCISE		EXERCISE + CO2
0	639.8	0	757.4
8	354.7	9	411.24
17	515.6	17	222.7
23	293.0	25	230.7
61	213.2*	63	173.8**

Comparison to rest value * $p<0.05$, ** $p<0.01$.

These data show that at increased work rates the EBI reduces significantly when compared to lower work rates. This is consistent with our previous hypothesis that breathing pattern during early exercise is predominately under behavioural control and that the increased metabolic demand with increasing exercise overrides this. The ventilatory response therefore, becomes more physiological at higher work rates with reduced behavioural control.

MODIFICATION OF CHEMORESPONSIVENESS

Hypocapnia as a result of idiopathic hyperventilation may affect breathing pattern in other ways. We hypothesised that chronic hypocapnia in patients with idiopathic hyperventilation may cause the central chemoreceptors to be reset to a lower CO_2 threshold. This could explain the augmented ventilatory response to normocapnic exercise and apparent intolerance of a physiological CO_2 level described above. We have studied CO_2 sensitivity in patients with idiopathic hyperventilation at rest and found that it is within the normal range. The mean (SD) CO_2 sensitivity in 30 patients with idiopathic hyperventilation was 1.52(0.6) l/min/mmHg. The normal range is usually quoted at 1.5 to 4.0 l/min/mmHg. Amongst this population of patients with idiopathic hyperventilation there were several subjects with CO_2 sensitivities below the normal range.

We therefore postulated that despite the slope of the CO_2 ventilatory response being within the normal range, patients with idiopathic hyperventilation have altered CO_2 control point on exercise. In other words, although the rise in ventilation per unit rise in arterial CO_2 is normal, this rise may start at a lower level of CO_2.

This pattern has been demonstrated previously by Zandbergen in 1991[19]. He showed that in a group of panic disorder patients the CO_2 sensitivity measured as the slope of the CO_2 ventilatory response was similar to a control group, however this response line in panic attack patients was shifted to the left by 5 mmHg compared to the control group.

Other groups have also been shown to have abnormal CO_2 responses. Athletes [20], breath-hold divers [21], submarine escape instructors [22] and underwater hockey players [23] have been reported to have reduced CO_2 responsiveness. Such alterations in physiology may be related to many factors including training, behavioural and cognitive factors and in some circumstances by sensations of pain and discomfort as in various disease states. The finding that in breath-hold divers the CO_2 response returns towards normality during periods away from work, supports the concept that the alterations in physiology may be adaptive rather than genetically determined.

Alteration of CO_2 sensitivity is thought to be a feature of endurance training and in some studies endurance trained cyclists have been demonstrated to have reduced CO_2 responsiveness in some studies as compared to normals [20]. It has been suggested that this may be mediated through altered CO_2 sensitivity however the literature to date on this subject is inconsistent and conflicting.

In an attempt to demonstrate altered chemoresponsiveness we have studied 8 patients with idiopathic hyperventilation 4 males, 4 females mean age (SD) 53.4 (7) years, 10 endurance trained cyclists (10 males, mean (SD) 23.8 (7)) and compared them to 8 male normal controls mean age 23.1(5) years.

We demonstrated that CO_2 sensitivity (rate of rise in ventilation per unit rise in $PetCO_2$) at rest was within the normal range in all 3 groups using a CO_2 rebreathe test [24]. Mean (SD) CO_2 sensitivity was 2.4 (0.4) l/min/mmHg in the cyclists, and 3.02(0.99) l/min/mmHg in the control group. The mean (SD) CO_2 sensitivity at rest for a large group of patients with idiopathic hyperventilation as discussed above was 1.52 (0.6) l/min/mmHg. All subjects then performed a maximal cardio-respiratory exercise test on a cycle ergometer and a steady state exercise test at 30 % of maximal work rate achieved on their maximal tests. The steady state test was performed under hyperoxic conditions to allow us to study central chemoreceptor responses in isolation. During the exercise test, once steady state was achieved, 100% oxygen was titrated into the inspired limb of the biased flow circuit described above. A new steady state was then accomplished in approximately 4-6 minutes under hyperoxic conditions and then CO_2 was also added to the inspired limb of the biased flow circuit by the inflow step wise technique [25] to hypercapnic levels. Control point was estimated using the mean of 2 independent investigators as the point at which ventilation began to rise in a linear fashion during CO_2 replacement.

Maximal $PetCO_2$ at test termination was significantly lower in patients with idiopathic hyperventilation compared to controls (mean (SD) $PetCO_2$ 53.5(4.3) mmHg versus 62.6 (4.8)mmHg ($p<0.01$)).

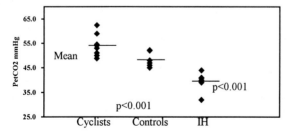

Fig 4. Central Control Point Derived From Hyperoxic Hypercapnic Steady State Exercise Tests in Cyclists, Controls and patients with Idiopathic Hyperventilation (IH)

The mean (SD) control point in patients with idiopathic hyperventilation was 39.7 (3.4)mmHg compared to 47.8(2.8)mmHg in the control group (normal range 45 ±0.82). This difference was highly significant (p<0.001). The mean (SD) control point in cyclists was 54.1(4.1), which was significantly higher than that of both the idiopathic hyperventilation and control groups.

These data would suggest that although the ventilatory response due to the CO_2 sensitivity is not altered from the control group, patients with idiopathic hyperventilation have a significantly lower CO_2 control point. This confirms that the ventilatory response to CO_2 in this group is shifted to the left and therefore occurs at a lower CO_2 level. This altered chemoresponsiveness at least partially explains the apparent intolerance of the physiological level of CO_2 during CO_2 replacement.

This finding of altered control point for CO_2 may not be the only explanation for the inappropriate level of ventilation seen on exercise in these individuals. We investigated the effect of performing work, with and without CO_2 replacement to normocapnic levels. We investigated 16 patients with idiopathic hyperventilation (10 females, mean (SD) age 55(12) years). All subjects performed hypocapnic and normocapnic maximal cycle ergometer exercise tests. During freewheel, there was no significant difference in ventilation between hypocapnic and normocapnic tests i.e. the addition of CO_2 did not exaggerate the ventilatory response to unloaded exercise. However at 40 watts of exercise, replacement of CO_2 to normocapnic levels provoked a further ventilatory response when compared to hypocapnic exercise at this level. Mean (SD) minute ventilation at 40 watts during normocapnic exercise was 53(17) l/min, compared with 34(13) l/min during hypocapnic exercise. This would suggest that the inappropriate increase in ventilation seen in patients with idiopathic hyperventilation on exercise may be the result of an interaction between performing work and the addition of CO_2. The mechanism of this is not clear. Endogenous CO_2 production from exercising muscles may stimulate this via the altered chemoresponsiveness discussed above. However other mechanisms may be at play, including altered perception of effort and dyspnoea during exercise or an interaction with sensory input from muscles performing work. The effect of emotional and behavioural factors on altered control point were investigated to observe whether anxiety levels (as measured by HADs score) were related to altered chemostasis. Although there was a significant negative correlation of $PetCO_2$ during hyperoxic steady state exercise and anxiety r = -0.797 (p<0.05), we have not been able to demonstrate a correlation between control point and anxiety although numbers studies thus far may not be sufficient to demonstrate significance.

SUMMARY

Idiopathic hyperventilation is therefore the name given to a condition of unknown aetiology which causes symptoms commonly presenting to chest clinics. Subjects with this condition demonstrate inappropriate levels and variability of ventilation especially during low work-rate exercise (such as walking). This response is thought to be caused by behavioural influences. In this chapter we have discussed quantification of this inappropriate breathing pattern and the effects on this of altering carbon dioxide levels. Carbon dioxide replacement to physiological levels produces an even more exaggerated rise in ventilation during exercise. Further studies on our patients have shown that this at least in part may be due to an alteration in central chemoreceptor control point to CO_2 and we postulate that intolerance to endogenous CO_2 production from exercising muscles may contribute to this exaggerated ventilatory response. Carbon dioxide replacement also appears to reduce variability in ventilation. Once more as a result of reduced CO_2 control point this is brought about by an increased drive to breathe thus reducing behavioural aspects of the ventilatory pattern.

We feel that initially the response to exercise in patients with idiopathic hyperventilation is caused by the anxiety which is known to be associated with this condition. As this response becomes more chronic, chemoresponsiveness is altered and the abnormal ventilatory response to exercise becomes both "physiological" for that patient and a conditioned response. Retraining in breathing pattern potentially therefore may reverse these changes and offers hope for a "cure" for this condition.

REFERENCE LIST

1. DaCosta J.M. (1871) On irritable heart: a clinical study of a form of functional cardiac disorder and its consequences. Amer. J. med Sci 61:17–52.
2. Haldane J. S. and Poulton E. P. (1908). The effect of the want of oxygen on respiration. J. Physiol. 37:390–407.
3. Collip J. B. and Backus P. L. (1920) The effect of prolonged hyperpnoea in carbon dioxide combining power of plasma, the carbon dioxide tension of alvelolar air and the excretoion of acid and basic phosphate and ammonium by the kidneys. Amer. J. Physiol.;51:568-579.
4. White P. D. and Hahn R. G. (1929) The symptoms of sighing in cardiovascular diagnosis. Amer. J. med Sci. 177:179–188.
5. Thompson W. P. (1943) The electrocardiogram in the hyperventilation syndrome. Amer Heart J. 25:372–390.
6. Soley M. H. and N. W. Shock. (1938) The etiology of effort syndrome. Amer. J. med Sci. 196: 840–852.
7. Lowry T. P. (1967) Hyperventilation and hysteria. Springfield, III, Charles C. Thomas
8. Lum C. (1976) The syndrome of habitual chronic hyperventilation. In: Modern trends in psychosomatic medicine. O. W. Hill ed. Bitterwoth publ, London; 11: pp196-230
9. Ley R. (1991) The effect of breathing retraining and the centrality of hyperventilation in panic disorder a reinterpretation of experimental findings. Behavioural Res. & Ther 29: 301-304.
10. Hornsveld H.K, Garssen B, Fiedeldij Dop M.J.C, Spiegel van P.I, and Haes J.C.J.M. (1996) Double – blind placebo – controlled study of the hyperventilation provocation test and validity of the hyperventilation. Lancet. 348:154–58.
11. Dixhoorn J. van. Duivenvoorden H. J. (1985) Efficacy of Nijmegen questionnaire in recognition of the hyperventilation syndrome. J. Psychosom. Res., 29: 199-206
12. Folgering H, Jongmans M, Cox N, Dekhuijzen P. (1991) Treatment of hyperventilation during pulmonary rehabilitation. Eur. Respir. J. 4 Suppl 14, 222S
13. Howell J. B. L. (1997) The hyperventilation syndrome: a syndrome under threat? Thorax, 52 (Suppl 3): S30–S34.
14. Plum F. (1970) Neurological itegration of behavioural and metabolic control of breathing. In: Porter R, ed. Breathing: Hering – Breuer Centenary Symposium. Churchill, London pp159–81.
15. Masokoa Y. and Homma I. (1999) Expiratory time determined by individual anxiety levels in humans. J. Appl Physiol, 86 (4): 1329–1336.
16. Datta A. K. Shea S. A. Horner R. L. Guz A. (1991) The influence of induced hypocapnia and sleep on the endogenous respiratory rhythm in humans. Jour of Physiol. 440:17–33.
17. Morgan N. and Cameron I. R. (1984) Respiratory response to behavioural and metabolic stimulation Clin. Sci. 67 (Suppl 9): 61 p.
18. Cherniack NS, von Euler C, Homma I and Kao FF. (1956) Experimentally induced cheyne – stokes breathing Respir Physiol 187:395–398.
19. Zandbergen J. Aalst V Van, Loof C. de, Pols H. Griez E. (1991) No hyperventilation in panic disorder. Psychiatry Res.39: 13–19.
20. McConnell A.K. and Semple E.S.G. (1996) Ventilatory sensitivity to carbon dioxide: the influence of exercise and athleticism. Med Sci. Sports Exerc. 28 (6) 685–691.
21 Rahn H, editor. (1965) Physiology of breath-hold diving and the Ama of Japan. NAS – NRC publication 1341, Washington, DC: National Academy of Science.
21. Schaeffer K. E. (1965) Adaptation to breath-hold diving. In Rahn H, ed Physiology of breath hold diving and Ama of Japan. NAS – NRC publication 1341 Washington DC: National academy of Science 237–252.

22. Davis F. M. Graves M. P. Guy J. B., Prisk K.and Tanner T. E. (1987) Carbon dioxide and breath hold times in underwater hockey players. Undersea Biomed Res, 14(6) 527–534
23. Read D.J.C. (1967) A clinical method for assessing the ventilatory response to carbon dioxide. Australian Annals of Medicine 16: 20-32.
24. Cummin A.R.C. Alison J. Jacobi S. Iyawe V. I. and Saunders K. B. (1986) Ventilatory sensitivity to inhaled carbon dioxide around the control point during exercise. Clinical Science, 71:17–22.

The Art of Breathing in the East and the West

Effects of the Eastern Art of Breathing

Yutaka Haruki and Hiroki Takase
School of Human Sciences, Waseda University, 2 -579-15 Mikajima, Tokorozawa, Saitama 359-1192, JAPAN

Summary: This chapter outlines the Eastern art of breathing and introduces a preliminary experiment related to breathing art involving bending and stretching of the legs. First, the ideological and cultural backgrounds of the Eastern art of breathing are summarized and ideas common to different types of the Eastern art of breathing are touched upon. Specifically, the paper refers to implications of the mind and the body in the art of breathing and stresses the importance of abdominal breathing and exhaling with a slow rhythm. Furthermore, the effects of the art of breathing involving physical movements are outlined. These effects include activation of blood circulation, stretching and relaxation of the muscles, graceful postures and movements, arousal of physical sensations, awareness of mood, image inducement, control of behavior and an understanding of certain things within one's entire physical system.

The paper then alludes to the art of breathing which teaches how to breathe while doing leg stretching and bending. It also reports a preliminary experiment related to the effects of breathing art on blood circulation and changes in mood. A study comparing a slow and a fast tempo exercise is presented with preliminary results showing that different speeds cause various changes in the total amount of hemoglobin in the blood, as well as changes in mood. However, further research is required to determine whether these changes are a result of breathing.

Key words: Eastern breathing art, Emotion, Blood circulation

According to James-Lange's theory, all emotions accompany some kind of "physical changes" and change in blood circulation is commonly observed as one of such changes (caused by change in muscle activities) [1]. In the East, on the other hand, the mind and the body are always considered as one and inseparable. It is obvious from this that James-Lange's theory concides with the pattern of Eastern thoughts. This paper will take up the effects of the art of breathing on the mind and the body. Firstly, its theory, essentials and effects will be explained. Further, the results of an ongoing preliminary experiment performed on the effects of the art of breathing involving the bending and stretching of legs, will be demonstrated.

I. Ideas and Cultures Behind the Eastern Art of Breathing

It is an indisputable fact that breathing is the most important physical response for sustenance of life. One could go on living for a month without any food and for a week without water. However, if breathing is stopped, life could not go on even for a few minutes.

The breathing response is automatically maintained by an automatic nervous system as with reflexes of other internal organs. Unlike such reflexes of other internal organs, however, a breathing response is controlled by the somatic nervous system as well. In other words, breathing can be done either unconsciously or consciously. Since breathing is essential for the sustenance of life, it takes the form of a double circuit.

People in general, either in the West or in the East, have very little interest in breathing. One of the reasons is probably because air is available for free while food and water cost money.

There seems to have existed in ancient times some knowledge about a breathing art in the Western culture, but its importance probably ceased around the Middle Ages. In contrast, knowledge about a breathing art has existed all along in the Eastern culture and the difference can probably be explained by different ideological backgrounds of the two cultures [2] [3].

1) Holistic Theory

The present day Western culture seems to have a theory that a human being consists of body and mind, that the body, considered to be a substance like a machine, is different from the mind. In Eastern culture, however, a theory separating the body and the mind in a clear-cut manner never developed. It has always been the predominant idea in Eastern culture that the mind is closely linked to physical conditions and that physical conditions are closely linked to the mind. The point of the theory is that the two are linked to each other so closely that they are inseparable. It is because of this theory that there has not developed in the Eastern culture any technology such as Western medicine as a science.

Behind the phenomenal success of today's Western medicine may be the fact the Western medicine separated mind and body and completely isolated one from the other. However it is probably because of this theory that the Western culture has a lack of knowledge about the Eastern Art of breathing. Regarding the body as something like a machine seems to have created the tendency to focus only on the breathing reflex and not on the fact that breathing can be done consciously. As another possible cause of the phenomenon, the Western theory that breathing is done mechanically brushed aside the inconceivable idea that the mind has something to do with breathing. Eastern culture theorizes that the mind and the body are invariably linked to each other and based on this theory, special attention has been focused on the fact that while breathing is a mechanical reflex, it is also a mental response.

Those specialized in modern medicine are loath to think that the mind has something to do with the body, but some have recently come to recognize the importance of the interrelationship between these two as seen in the emergence of psychosomatic medicine or behavioral medicine, for instance. As a result, there will probably be a growing interest in breathing and a breathing art.

2) Breathing as a cause

Western culture is distinct from Eastern culture in that it separates mind and body and values the mind. As opposed to this, Eastern culture values both the mind and the body without separating them. In other words, if you think about the causal relationship between mind and body, Western culture tends to think of the mind first and then the body. It is not necessarily the case with Eastern culture where mind and body are considered to be related dynamically. This difference seems to account for the different attitudes toward breathing between the two cultures. For instance, when physiological psychologists consider the relationship between the mind and breathing, they consider the mind to be an independent variable (cause) and breathing to be a dependent variable (result). As an illustration, consider the case where a stressed mind causes breathing to be shallower [4][5]. Though this is a fact, the art of breathing is not an outgrowth of this notion. The concept of a breathing art results from focusing on a causal relationship that breathing changes the state of mind. Breathing is at once a result and a cause of something. If a breathing response is simply part of all physical reflexes and has nothing to do with the mind, it would be hard to think of the art of breathing. The fact that breathing can be done consciously leads to the development of a breathing art.

3) Breathing and Japanese culture

Breathing arts originated in India and China, and probably existed in Greece and Persia as well. The Japanese culture was influenced by Indian and Chinese cultures through Buddhism. In particular, Zen Buddhism brought by Dogen, a Zen priest who studied in China in the 1220s, had an immeasurable influence on the Japanese culture later on. Dogen established Japan's own Zen Buddhism. This Zen Buddhism became the core of Japan's unique culture. Zen meditation, which is practiced by way of training one's mind, is regarded as the most important part of all Zen Buddhism. What is considered to be the key factor in Zen meditation is a breathing art. For this reason Japan manifested interest from early on in the relations between breathing and the mind. Zen Buddhism has bred Japan's unique culture and was instrumental in turning into spiritual artful forms those martial arts, tea ceremonies and other day-to-day manners. This explains the fact that the importance of breathing has been recognized with respect to all art activities in Japan (e.g., calligraphy). It seems to be the prevalent idea in the Japanese culture that a breathing art and spirituality cannot be completely separated from each other. In other words, it has practically become a matter of common knowledge that a breathing art is deeply related to the building of mind. Japan has introduced several breathing arts and has zealously imported some from India and China probably because of the foregoing theories and traditions.

II. Essentials of Eastern Art of Breathing

There are many breathing arts. As stated below, a breathing art does not exist as an independent technique but is interrelated to all forms of Eastern techniques (physical movements and manipulation of the mind). Consequently, the Yoga breathing art is known in India and the Qigong and Taijiquan breathing arts are known in China. In Japan, as stated earlier, the Zen breathing art is well known. As you can see from this, there are numerous breathing arts involving their respective unique techniques. However, they all have common qualities as the Eastern arts of breathing [6].

1) Body regulation, breathing regulation and mind regulation

Body regulation means the control of one's posture and body movements. Breathing regulation means control of breathing. Mind regulation means management of the condition of consciousness. In accordance with an Eastern holistic idea, everything about the mind and the body must be manipulated in a dynamic way in order to control the condition of one's mind and body.

For the practice of "Gyo" (Eastern mind/body training method) , which aims at control of the mind and the body, the key words are body regulation, breathing regulation and mind regulation.   For instance, control of the mind alone would be inadequate if there is something wrong with the body.   Control of the body and breathing is considered important as well as control of the mind.

What should be noted here is the fact that breathing control is involved in control of the mind and the body and that a breathing art is part of the "Gyo" practice.   Incidentally, "breathing" can also be translated into "息" (breath) in Japanese.   The Chinese character "息" is known as a compound word made of "鼻" (nose) and "心" (mind).   In other words, in China and in Japan it has been understood that breathing is not only a physical response but a mental response as well.

As seen from this, a breathing art is essential for regulation of mind and body by putting them together.   It is to be noted, however, that a breathing art could not exist without regulation of mind and body.   It needs to be understood that these three are interrelated with one another dynamically.   This is the reason, as referred to earlier, that a breathing art does not exist by itself but as a constituent part of the "Gyo" practice.

2) Importance of abdominal breathing

A breathing response has many properties.   It is particularly so with conscious breathing, and this may be the reason for the existence of numerous breathing arts.   For instance, such properties include inhaling and exhaling, chest breathing and abdominal breathing, long breathing and short breathing, and breathing through the nose and breathing through the mouth.

In the East, abdominal breathing is advocated. Specifically, abdominal breathing involves movements of the diaphragm.   When you inhale, the diaphragm contracts and comes down.   A swelling abdomen can be observed from the outside.   Physiologically, this breathing method is considered effective.   There is also a theory that the pressure of up and down movements of the diaphragm on the internal organs activates blood circulation.

More importantly, abdominal breathing has psychological effects.   As everyone knows through their day to day experiences, when you are feeling insecure or stressed, there is a tendency to breathe with the chest and breathing tends to be shallow [7][8]. If breathing is done with the abdomen in such a case, some easing of your stress is experienced.   Since the mechanism of interactions between abdominal breathing and psychological aspects is not clear, it is necessary to confirm such a mechanism in the future.

3) Importance of exhaling

Breathing reflexes consist of inhaling and exhaling.   This can be done consciously as well.   This raises a question of which breathing reflex should be considered more important. The Eastern arts of breathing attaches more importance to exhaling.

It teaches that if you exhale air with a conscious effort against the air pressure and then relax, air enters your body automatically. The theory states that the more you let air out of your lungs, the larger will be the amount of air you inhale.

As for psychological effects of these breathing methods, exhaling is known to be more relaxing.   There are data to the effect that under a tense situation the interval between exhalation and inhalation becomes shorter [9][10][11].   According to the paradigm that breathing is a cause, a brief pause following long exhalation is helpful for your relaxation.   Physiologically, inhalation is interrelated with sympathetic nervous activity and exhalation with parasympathetic nervous activity, a theory which is consistent with psychological effects.

4) Slow rhythm

It is said that normally one breathes about fourteen times a minute.   However, it has been observed that under a tense situation one's breathing becomes shallow and fast.   The Eastern arts of breathing advocates breathing with a slow rhythm.   A veteran Zen priest is known to breathe two or three times a minute.   A slow rhythm means a long and slow exhalation and prolongation of the interval between each exhalation and inhalation.

III. Effects of Eastern Art of Breathing

The Eastern art of breathing practiced for mind and body regulation does not involve breathing alone as explained earlier.   In numerous cases, it involves mind and body regulation. To put it differently, any breathing art is only part of the "Gyo" practice.   Consequently, the effects of the Eastern art of breathing are hardly distinguishable from the effects of the "Gyo" practice.   Therefore, I am going to speak about the effects of practicing "Gyo".

As for the effects of "Gyo", sufficient scientific studies are regrettably not being conducted at this time.   In recent years data have appeared with respect to physiological and psychological effects of Zen meditation, Yoga and Qigong, but they are far from sufficient. This means there is a lack of a general view concerning the effects of "Gyo".   However, there are many Gyo-related traditions which have been handed down from India, China and Japan. They can be summarized as follows [12]:

1) Activation of blood circulation

Prelimary experiments show that repetition of conscious breathing accompanied by slow bending and leg stretching movements as in Taijiquan causes sweating and activates blood circulation although Gyo is not as vigorous as most sports.

2) Relaxation of muscles

The "Gyo" practice aims at relaxation of the mind and the body by restoring a total balance between the two through repetitious stretching and relaxing of the muscles.   Yoga is typical of "Gyo".

3) Graceful posture and movements

A long time scale movement of the body is one of the achievements aimed at by "Gyo", that is, to make body movements graceful including the movements of limbs.   Yoga and Taijiquan, arts which regulate the balance of posture and movements, are based on a theory that through such practice, graceful posturing and movements can help promote and maintain a balance of mental activities.

4) Arousal of physical senses

Body movements involved in the practice of "Gyo" are not aimed at hardening the muscles as in sports. Such body movements are to cause a muscular sensation (proprioceptive stimulation) thereby arousing physical sensations. While the five senses of a human being relate to stimulation coming from outside (exteroceptive stimulation), a muscular sensation or a movement sensation is self-caused. The five senses cause a person to experience something from outside which stimulates the senses. A muscular movement or a movement sensation makes one experience oneself. In other words, it can be said that the arousal of physical sensations is the arousal of the sensation of being alive.

5) Awareness of mood

A mood forms the basis of mental activities. It is linked to physical sensations and the five senses. The "Gyo" practice attempts to regulate mood and enhances the awareness of it. It is through enhancement of the awareness of mental activities and regulation of a mood that higher mental activities can be stabilized and activated.

6) Image inducement

Images are the basis of cognition. They are made up of physical sensations, the five senses and memories. It can be said that colorful images make for fertile mental activities. Movements based on the "Gyo" practice are instrumental in activating images.

7) Control of behavior

If the practice of "Gyo" help to control behavior, it will no doubt be helpful in our day-to-day living. According to health psychologists, a good lifestyle (living habits) is imperative for the maintenance and improvement of health, and "Gyo", if practiced daily, would be helpful in forming a healthy lifestyle.

8) Understanding of one's whole system

The relationship between "Gyo" and higher mental activities is unknown at this point in time. However, one interesting question has been posed.

Japanese culture attaches importance to understanding not only what is logical but also what is beyond logic. The Japanese word "wakaru" (understand) means to understand something in a logical sense. However, to understand something which is beyond a logical sense means to understand something "within one's whole system." "System" means the body (direct experiences). As this illustration shows, true understanding of something requires involvement of the body. Eastern thoughts do not separate the mind and the body. Consequently, Eastern thoughts may suggest that higher mental activities involve the body. However, further studies need to be conducted in this regard in the future.

The effects produced by the practice of "Gyo" have been presented. It may be said that breathing relates to all things. However, breathing, in particular, may involve the factors described in 1) through 5). Breathing is believed to produce physiological effects and help control the basis of mental activities.

According to the "Gyo" practice, smooth blood circulation is essential for a healthy mind and body. From a physiological point of view, firstly one must have good circulation of blood as mentioned in 1). Secondly, there is a matter of moods. According to Eastern thoughts, "ki" or "qui" is the most important concept, however mood will be focused on here. A good mood means an uninhibited and comfortable mood. This can probably be attained through the practice of "Gyo" as described in 2) through 5). To activate one's mind and body is to relax them. A preliminary experiment was conducted to find out about relaxation of the mind and the body; the following is an outline of the findings.

IV. Physiological and psychological effects of the art of breathing involving leg bending and stretching[1]

Taijiquan is unique in that one moves from one place to another with his/her legs bent and waist lowered. The main part of the art as exercise is leg stretching and bending. Moreover, the essential part is not to do stretching as in walking, sports and ballet dancing but to do bending. As for breathing, basically one exhales when bending and inhales when stretching and this is done with a rhythm. These movements are believed to activate the muscles of the femoral region and activate blood circulation in the legs. Particularly, blood in the legs on its way to the heart (blood in veins) tends to be stagnant but leg stretching and bending is believed to activate blood circulation.

Taijiquan is different from other sports in that it involves slow movements and provokes our deep interest in the effects Taijiquan may have on the mind and the body.

The purpose of our experiment was to determine the effects of leg stretching and bending and breathing on blood circulation and moods. For this purpose "Qishi", the first movement of Taijiquan was employed. "Qishi" is a movement involving the bending of legs and lowering the body while exhaling and involving the stretching of the legs, getting up and inhaling. This process was repeated. The effects of the speed of these movements were also examined.

1) Method

Fifteen students of a women's physical education college in Tokyo participated in the experiment. They had no impediments in breathing or locomotive organs.

Blood circulation in the legs was examined by fitting each subject with a NIRO MONITOR (NIRO-300, Hamamatsu Hotonics) on the Vastus lateralis muscle; the quantities of oxygenated and deoxygenated hemoglobin in the blood in the legs were measured following leg bending and stretching. Oxygenated hemoglobin and deoxygenated hemoglobin combined are the total amount of hemoglobin and blood volume index. In order to examine the psychological changes, an SD (semantic differential) method and POMS (Profile of Mood States) tests were conducted to examine the emotional condition of each subject before and after bending and stretching. These tests were carried out on the basis of the following formula: Stretching and bending speeds (slow and fast) × between each set (1st set -10th set) × within a set (pre-exercise, exercise).

[1] The experiment was conducted at Research Institute of Physical Fitness, Japan Woman,s College of Physical Education. We thank Atsuko Kagaya.Ph.D and Yoshiho Muraoka.Ph.D for their help.

As for the procedures, the subjects were asked to stand up following their replies to POMS and SD tests. After confirming that the blood in their legs was in a stabilized condition, they were asked to stretch and bend their legs with controlled breathing by keeping time to a metronome set at a slow tempo (0.15/sec.) or a fast tempo (0.5/sec.). During their exercise, the work of collecting physiological data (data on their movements) was carried out. The leg stretching and bending exercise with controlled breathing took place for ten trials. After the exercise, the subjects were asked to sit down and rest for one minute while checking the SD test. With ten trials counted as a set, ten sets (100 trials) were carried out. The subject had a one-minute rest between each set. Following the completion of ten sets, the subjects underwent POMS.

2) Results
a. Data on physiological index

An analysis of variance was conducted with respect to three factors speed (S/F)× between each set (1st set -10th sets)×within a set (pre-exercise, exercise) with the total amount of hemoglobin as a dependent variable. According to the findings, exercise with a fast speed resulted in a significant decrease in the total amount of hemoglobin between the pre-exercise and the exercise. On the other hand, a slow speed exercise showed no significant hemogrobin change between the pre-exercise and the exercise. Furthermore, a slow speed exercise resulted in a greater increase in the total amount of hemoglobin during the exercise (see Figs. 1 and 2) than in the case of a fast speed exercise. This result is significant from a statistical point of view.

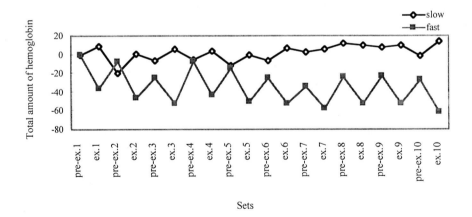

Fig.1. Total amount of hemoglobin of each set

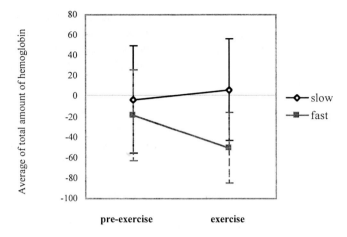

Fig.2. Average total amount of hemoglobin in pre-exercise and exercise

b. Data on psychological index

There were statistically significant differences between the two movement speeds in each item "vivacious - anemic," "relaxed - tense," "active - quiet," and "ongoing - meditative." In other words, slow movements were seemingly more lively, tense, active, and ongoing than fast movements.

As for the results of POMS, an analysis of the following six subordinate scales shows that "stress (anxiety),""depression," and "confusion" were significantly different before and after ten sets. This shows that with the passage of time during the exercise of ten sets, tense and depressed moods or a confused state of mind subsided.

3) Discussion
a. Physiological effects

The results show that when stretching and bending the legs while exhaling at a fast speed, the amount of blood in the femoral region of the legs decreased and in the case of exercise at a slow speed, there was a slight, not significant, increase, in the average amount of blood in the femoral region.

It is generally believed that when engaged in dynamic sports, the amount of blood in the muscles functioning at the time increases for the supply of oxygen. However, the results show that when stretching and bending legs while exhaling at a fast speed, the opposite is the case. Namely, the amount of blood in the muscles functioning during the exercise decreases. According to the raw data of the time series on the amount of blood (the total amount of hemoglobin) with respect to a subject who did leg stretching and bending at a fast speed, the amount of blood decreased immediately after the subject started to exercise and several seconds later (about seven or ten seconds), the amount of blood began to increase. This is also verified by the time series related to the amount of blood of the majority of subjects who exercised at a slow speed.

In this experiment, the number of trials in a set was the same for both the fast tempo exercise and the slow tempo exercise. As a result, the amount of time required for a set was different between the slow and the fast tempo exercises. The result of the experiment shows that the amount of blood decreased in the case of the fast tempo exercise and that the amount of blood increased in the case of the slow tempo exercise. This is probably because in the case of a fast tempo exercise, the amount of time required for the exercise was comparatively short and the exercise came to an end before the amount of blood was brought back to a higher level; in the case of the slow tempo exercise, the amount of time required for the exercise was comparatively long thus allowing the amount of blood to be brought back to a higher level.

It has been verified through these results that the amount of blood in the femoral region, the muscles which function while performing leg stretching and bending, undergoes a dynamic change. There are few data on the amount of blood measured at the time of exercise and at the present stage where a series of experiments need to be conducted with various factors as independent variables, our experiment may represent a firm step forward in a new direction.

Leg stretching and bending has been found to cause a dynamic change in blood particularly around the muscles of the femoral region. Given the fact that blood circulation is highly essential for appropriate supply of oxygen to active muscles and that such oxygen will smoothly enter blood vessels from outside through controlled breathing, there is a greater possibility that leg stretching and bending combined with controlled breathing is effective in activating blood circulation and facilitating the supply of oxygen to the system.

b. Psychological effects

After a ten-set exercise, tense and depressed moods as well as a confused state of mind (POMS test) were seen to have subsided compared with those before the exercise. However, it should not be readily concluded that this is a result of leg stretching and bending with controlled breathing because the change may be attributed to the fact that a subject got accustomed to doing the exercise. Furthermore, confirmation is required in this respect. The results of the SD scale seem inconsistent with our understanding of speed. However, leg stretching and bending combined with controlled breathing as done in this experiment is something we seldom experience. Therefore, this seeming inconsistency observed in this experiment may not be an inconsistency but a special effect of such an exercise.

Taijiquan which is part of the practice of "Gyo" is far from daily routine. Taijiquan is believed to produce better blood and "Qi" circulation. As for blood circulation, the results of this experiment are believed to have verified to a certain extent that leg stretching and bending is effective in improving blood circulation. As for "Qi" (good mood based on the SD scale and POMS), however, no tangible results were obtained. Further experimental research work is needed.

REFERENCES

1. Cornelius RR (1996) The Science of Emotion. Prentice-Hall, Inc.
2. Bankart CP, Koshikawa F, Nedate K & Haruki, Y (1992) When West meets East: contributions of Eastern traditions to the future of psychotherapy. Psychotherapy 29:141-149
3. Bankart CP (1997) Talking cures: A history of Western & Eastern psychotherapies. Books/Cole Publishing Company
4. Boiten F, Frijda NH, Wientjes JC (1994) Emotions and respiratory patterns: Review and critical analysis. International Journal of Psychophysiology 17:103-128
5. Grossman P (1983) Respiration, stress and cardiovascular function. Psychophysiology 20:284-300
6. Haruki Y, Homma I (eds) (1996) How to breathe. Asahi Newspaper Company, Tokyo (Iki no shikata. Asahi shinnbunnsya)
7. Ancoli S, Kamiya J (1979) Respiratory patterns during emotional expression. Biofeedback Self-regulation 4 :242
8. Ancoli S, Kamiya J, Ekman P (1980) Psychophysiological differentiation of positive and negative affects. Biofeedback Self-regulation 5:356-357
9. Cohen HD,Goodenough DR., Witkin HA, Oltman P, Gould H, Shulman E (1975) The effects of stress on components of the respiration cycle. Psychophysiology 12:377-380
10. Boiten FA (1993) Component analysis of task-related respiratory patterns. International Journal of Psychopysiology 15:91-104
11. Umezawa A (1991) Changes of respiratory activity during laboratory stress. Japanese Journal of Physiological Psychology and Psychophysiology 9:43-55 (Sutoresushigeki ni taisuru kokyuukatudou no henyou. Seirisinrigaku to seisinseirigaku)
12. Haruki Y (1998) Body Work as epistemology. Journal of Health Physical Education and Recreation Vol.48, 25:101-104 (Ninsikironn tositeno body work. Taiiku no kagaku)

BIOFEEDBACK FOR RESPIRATORY SINUS ARRHYTHMIA AND TANDEN BREATHING AMONG ZEN MONKS: STUDIES IN CARDIOVASCULAR RESONANCE

Paul Lehrer, PhD[1]

Department of Psychiatry
UMDNJ -- Robert Wood Johnson Medical School
671 Hoes Lane
Piscataway, New Jersey, 08854
USA

Summary: Resting heart rate is characterized by several overlapping oscillations at several frequencies. Oscillations at each frequency is related to a specific set of reflexes that plays a role in cardiovascular homeostasis. Recent research on biofeedback training to increase the amplitudes of these frequencies has found that people can accomplish this task by breathing at frequencies that resonate with oscillations at slower frequency ranges. The slower heart rate oscillations appear to reflect baroreflex activity. Such biofeedback training may exercise the baroreflexes and thereby increase baroreflex efficiency and decrease vulnerability to disorders characterized by autonomic hyperreactivity (e.g., asthma, hypertension, anxiety disorders). Zen monks have a low rate of cardiovascular disease, and also breathe very slowly during the practice of Zazen, causing resonance with oscillations in cardiovascular variables related to heart rate and blood pressure control. One very experienced monk breathed at a rate of approximately once/minute, and appeared to stimulate reflexes that control vascular tone and body temperature.

Key words: cardiac variability, respiratory psychophysiology, Zen, biofeedback

HEART RATE VARIABILITY

Heart rate among healthy people is known to be highly variable. In addition to showing great reactivity to psychologically or physically demanding tasks[1], it manifests a complex pattern of spontaneous overlapping oscillatory rhythms [2]. We have elsewhere outlined evidence for a theory that such oscillations represent homeostatic control mechanisms, and that the stability of almost any psychobiological system is maintained by reflexes reflected by these oscillations [3].

Fig. 1 shows cardiac variability of a normal individual at rest. Note that pattern of variability is irregular, but not random. Generally, greater complexity in this pattern reflects greater cardiovascular health and adaptability. Low levels of complexity in heart rate variability is associated with high risk of sudden cardiac death and/or cardiac infarction [4,5]. This pattern is composed of at least three superimposed frequencies. There is evidence that oscillations at each of these frequencies represents action of a particular set of reflexes involving autonomic control

[1]The author is indebted to the assistance of the following individuals in this research: Yuji Sakaki, Yoshihiro Saito, MA, Alexander Smetankin, PhD, Annabaker Garber, PhD, and Evgeny Vaschillo, PhD.

of the cardiovascular system, as will be outlined below. It is perhaps for this reason that complexity seems to reflect health of the system: greater complexity reflects a greater number of oscillating systems, hence better-modulated autonomic control, with more back-up systems. Amplitude of RSA has recently been found to be related to homeostatic capacity among human fetuses [6]; and high heart period variability and less blocking of this variability during mental challenge both have been found to be present among trained runners and individuals with naturally low heart rates [7]. Previous data have shown that cardiac variability is attenuated in emotional disorders such as panic disorder [8,9], generalized anxiety disorder [10], and depression [11]. It is depressed among at-risk infants [12]. It is thought to be a good index of autonomic balance during surgical anesthesia [13]. It is negatively correlated with age in an adult population [14], perhaps reflecting decline in homeostatic adaptability. It is positively associated with aerobic fitness [15], and it is a strong indicator of mortality from cardiac disease [16,17].

The overlapping three common adult heart rate oscillation frequencies can easily be seen in Fig 1, as follows:

1) High-frequency (fast) waves (.15-.4 Hz) . High-frequency heart rate oscillations are usually mediated by respiratory activity, which usually occurs within this frequency range in the normal adult population. Heart rate oscillations mediated by respiration are denoted as respiratory sinus arrhythmia (RSA), and are known to be vagally mediated [18,19,20] although there is some evidence that it reflects reflex actions that exert modulatory control over the parasympathetic system, rather than vagal tone per se. Porges [21] has pointed out that vagally-mediated cardiac decelerations often are accompanied by a *decrease* in RSA, This regularly occurs in the orienting reflex, when an individual is appraising a novel stimulus that has suddenly appeared. Porges suggests that heart rate decreases in this situation because modulatory influences over the cardio-vagal system suddenly decrease or stop, allowing a large vagal discharge. We should note that the high frequency band only reflects RSA when the individual actually breathes within this frequency range. When people breathe at a slower rate, the processes involved in mediating RSA may overlap with those mediating low-frequency waves (described below). RSA is produced by reflexes triggered by a number of respiratory-related factors, including intrathoracic pressure and chemical composition of the blood [2,22]. It also appears to be affected by rhythms generated within the CNS [23]

2) Low frequency (slow) waves (.05-.15 Hz). Heart rhythm fluctuations within this frequency range are usually under both sympathetic and parasympathetic control [24,25], although parasympathetic influences tend to be greater in the supine position. Rhythms in this range are highly correlated with baroreflex control, and may reflect baroreflex action [26], by which heart rate and blood pressure regulate each other. Vaschillo [27] has calculated that the baroreflex system is affected by an approximately 5-sec delay (probably due to vascular resistance), thus accounting for the peak of the low frequency rhythm at approximately 10 Hz in most individuals.

3) Very low frequency (very slow) waves (005-.05 Hz). Heart rhythm fluctuations within this frequency range are sympathetically controlled, and appear to be associated with internal control of vascular tone and body temperature [28,29,30]

Resonance, RSA biofeedback, and voluntary control of cardiac variability. Recent research on voluntary control of cardiac oscillation amplitudes shows that most individuals are able to increase the amplitudes of oscillations within the low and very low frequency ranges. In the case of the low-frequency range, one can easily demonstrate an increase in RSA amplitude when one

FIG 1. R-R Interval (RRI) from the electrocardiogram of a healthy individual during baseline conditions.

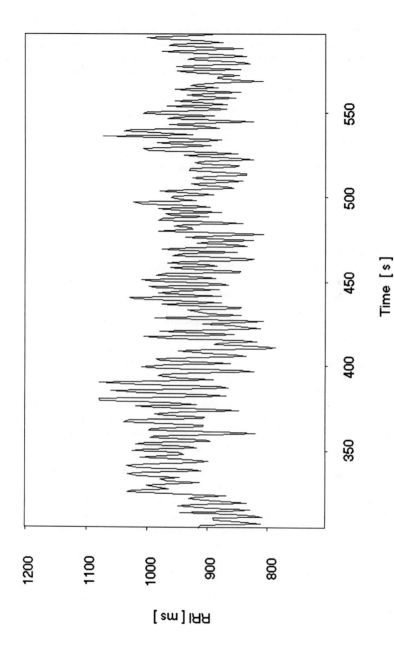

Note three overlapping oscillation patterns with periods of approximately 60 sec (very low frequency), 10 sec (low frequency), and 3-4 sec (high frequency).

breathes at the rate of approximately six times per minute. Vaschillo [31] has pointed out that, at this frequency, resonance occurs between processes ordinarily associated with high-frequency activity (i.e., RSA) and those associated with low-frequency activity (perhaps baroreflex control). The exact frequency at which resonance occurs for each individual may not be precisely 0.1 Hz (i.e., with a period of 6/min), but it occurs within the low-frequency range for almost everybody.

Vaschillo's studies involved having six healthy Russian cosmonauts sit before a computer-generated sine-wave, with another ray on the screen reflecting the subject's heart rate. The subject was instructed to match the computer-generated signal with the one that he controlled (although he was not informed that "his" signal reflected heart rate). Vaschillo [15] varied the frequency of oscillations through the low and very low-frequency ranges, and found the following in all subjects:

> 1) The highest amplitude heart rate oscillations were produced within the low-frequency range (averaging .1 Hz).

> 2) Oscillations in blood pressure also were affected by this task. The highest amplitude of blood pressure produced by this task was in the very low frequency range (approximately .03-0.05 Hz). Blood pressure oscillations were disorganized and at a low amplitude where heart rate oscillations were highest, and vice versa.

> 3) The heart rate and blood pressure oscillations at .1 Hz were 180° out of phase with each other, but were in phase at approximately .05 Hz.

Partially inspired by these findings, Russian investigators have utilized RSA biofeedback procedures to treat a number of disorders characterized by autonomic hyperreactivity, including asthma, hypertension, some cardiac arrhythmias, and anxiety disorders [32,33]. Russian researchers [20,21,34,35] have hypothesized that frequent production of regular high-amplitude heart rate oscillations at the same rate as oscillations produced by baroreflex activity acts to "exercise" the baroreflexes, and to make them more efficient. Increased homeostatic reflex efficiency, he further hypothesizes, is the mediating mechanism for the therapeutic effects of RSA biofeedback.

Although subjects in Vaschillo's studies did not seem to produce resonance entirely by respiratory maneuvers, it can easily be demonstrated that breathing at each individual's resonant frequency can produce very large increases in amplitude of RSA. In therapeutic protocols, trainees spontaneously tend to slow their respiration rates to within the frequency range of low-frequency HR variability. This occurred among all subjects in a small study from our laboratory of RSA biofeedback for treating asthma. In this study significant decreases occurred in respiratory impedance, both between- and within eight sessions of treatment.

CARDIAC VARIABILITY AMONG ZEN PRACTITIONERS WHILE PRACTICING TANDEN BREATHING

There is evidence that Zen practitioners have particularly low levels of serum lipids and low rates of cardiovascular disease [36], and also that they tend to spend many hours per day doing meditative exercises that usually involve breathing at very slow rates. It is possible that these individuals breathe at resonant frequencies, thus producing very high amplitudes of oscillations in heart rate, which, in turn, may produce similar effects to those of RSA biofeedback, and may, in part, account for the low rate of cardiovascular disease in this group. One particular discipline practiced during Zazen is that of "tanden breathing", where the individual deliberately focuses on each breath, and breathes slowly while thinking about an area of the body slightly below the navel.

To investigate the cardiac rhythm effects of tanden breathing, I undertook a study of cardiac variability among eleven Zen monks and nuns at various centers in Japan. The results of this study have been reported elsewhere [37], and will be summarized here.

The procedure was as follows: After attaching EKG electrodes to the wrists and strain gauge transducers around the chest, each individual was observed during six consecutive 5-min intervals: 1) a period of quiet sitting (breathing normally), 2) four contiguous 5-min periods of tanden breathing (with no break between them), followed by 3) a final period of quiet sitting.

For most subjects, we found that respiration rates fell to within the range associated with "low frequency" heart rate variability (.05-.15 Hz) during tanden breathing; and heart rate variability within this range correspondingly increased. Heart rate variability *decreased* within the high-frequency range (.15-.4 Hz), reflecting the shift in respiration rate (and hence RSA) from high frequency to slower waves. Total variability in heart rate also greatly increased.

Others have noted that, of the two great schools of Zen, practitioners of the Rinzai tradition tend to emphasize respiration more than those of the Soto tradition, and that Rinzai practitioners tend to breathe at a slower rates during practice of Zazen [38]. Our findings were similar. We also found a correspondingly higher amplitude of low-frequency heart oscillations among Rinzai than among Soto Zen participants. This result was statistically significant, despite the small number of individuals in this study.

One Rinzai master breathed approximately once/min and showed an increase in very low frequency waves (<.05 Hz). He also showed an increase in heart rate, and reported feeling warm during the period of Zazen, even though the room conditions were very cold. (The research took place during the month of January, and the room was unheated.)

These data are consistent with the theory that increased oscillation amplitude during slow breathing is caused by resonance between cardiac variability caused by respiration and that produced by physiological processes underlying slower rhythms. Usually the slow breathing and increased cardiac variability occurred within the low-frequency range, often associated with baroreflex action which, according to Vaschillo's findings, particularly reflects heart rate control. The extraordinarily slow breathing produced by the Rinzai master was within the very-low-frequency range of heart rate variability, and appeared to produce resonance with cardiovascular oscillations within within this range. The increased heart rate and sensations of warmth that occurred in this monk may have been caused by increased stimulation of autonomic reflexes associated with very low frequency heart rate variability.

CONCLUSIONS

Our data are consistent with the notion that Zen practitioners breathe at frequencies that produce resonance between rhythms of heart rate variability produced by breathing and those produced by autonomic regulatory reflexes. It is thus possible that these reflexes receive more exercise than usual in this population perhaps leading to exceptionally strong autonomic regulation among Zen monks. Further research will be necessary to determine whether the practice of tanden breathing bears a causal relationship with the low rate of cardiovascular disease in this group. If such a relationship is found, it is possible that some of the discipline involved in tanden breathing may be adapted for helping people who experience symptoms associated with autonomic dysregulation.

We also note that, whatever the cardiovascular effects of tanden breathing, it would be disrespectful to the Zen tradition to imply that these effects are the primary goal of practicing Zazen. The relationship between the respiratory and cardiac effects found in this study and the more subjective effects associated with spiritual growth have been investigated in a preliminary way. Early work on this topic has been summarized in a two-volume work edited by Akishige (1977).

REFERENCES

1. Schneiderman N, McCabe PM. (1989) Psychophysiological strategies in laboratory research. In: Schneiderman N, Weiss SM, Kaufman PG (Eds.), Handbook of research methods in cardiovascular behavioral medicine. Plenum, New York, Chapter 22, pp 349-364

2. Berntson GG, Caccioppo JT, Quigley KS (1993). Respiratory sinus arrhythmia: autonomic origins, physiological mechanisms, and psychophysiological implications. Psychophysiology 30:183-196

3. Giardino ND, Lehrer PM, Feldman JM (In press) The role of oscillations in self-regulation: their contribution to homeostasis. In: Kenny D, McGuigan FJ (eds) Stress and health: Research and clinical applications. Harwood publishers, Geneva

4. Goldberger A L, Rigney DR, Mietus J, Antman EM, Greenwald S (1988) Nonlinear dynamics in sudden cardiac death syndrome: Heart rate oscillations and bifurcations. Experientia 44:983-987

5. Kleiger RE, Miller J P, Bigger JT, Moss AJ (1987) Decreased heart rate variability and its association with increased mortality after acute myocardial infarction. American Journal of Cardiology 59:256-262.

6. Groome LJ, Loizou PC, Holland SB, Smith LA, Hoff C (1999) High vagal tone is associated with more efficient regulation of homeostasis in low-risk human fetuses. Developmental Psychobiology 35:25-34.

7. Boutcher SH, Nugent FW, McLaren PF, Weltman AL (1998) Heart period variability of trained and untrained men at rest and during mental challenge. Psychophysiology 35:16-22.

8. Asmundson GJG, Stein MB (1994) Vagal attenuation in panic disorder: An assessment of parasympathetic nervous system function and subjective reactivity to respiratory manipulations. Psychosomatic Medicine 56:187-193

9. Rechlin T, Weis M, Spitzer A, Kaschka WP (1994) Are affective disorders associated with alterations of heart rate variability? Journal of Affective Disorders 32:271-275.

10. Thayer JF, Friedman BH, Borkovec TD (1996) Autonomic characteristics of generalized anxiety disorder and worry. Biological Psychiatry 15:255-266

11. Yeragani VK, Balon R, Pohl R, Ramesh C (1995) Depression and heart rate variability. Biological Psychiatry 38:768-770

12. Rother M, Zwiener U, Eiselt M, Witte H, Zwacka G, Frenzel J (1987) Differentiation of healthy newborns and newborns-at-risk by spectral analysis of heart rate fluctuations and respiratory movements. Early Human Development 15:349-363.

13. Fleisher LA (1996) Heart rate variability as an assessment of cardiovascular status. Journal of Cardiothoracic Vascular Anesthesiology 10:659-671.

14. De Meersman RE (1993) Aging as a modulator of respiratory sinus arrhythmia. Journal of Gerontology 48:B74-B78

15. Sloan RP, DeMeersman RRE, Shapiro PA, Bagiella E, Chernikhova D, Kuhl JP, Paik M, Myers MM: Blood pressure variability responses to tilt are buffered by cardiac autonomic control. Am J Physiol 273 (Heart Circ Physiol 42): H1427-H1431, 1997.

16. Dougherty CM, Burr RL (1992) Comparison of heart rate variability in survivors and nonsurvivors of sudden cardiac arrest. American Journal of Cardioloby 70:441-448.

17. Huikuri HV, Makikallio TH, Airaksinen KE, Seppanen T, Puukka P, Raiha IJ, Sourander LB (1998) Power-law relationship of heart rate variability as a predictor of mortality in the elderly. Circulation 97:2031-2036

18. Porges SW (1986) Respiratory sinus arrhythmia: physiological basis, quantitative methods, and clinical implications. In: Grossman P, Janssen K, Vaitl D (eds) Cardiorespiratory and cardiosomatic psychophysiology. Plenum Press, New York

19. Grossman P, Wientjes K (1986) Respiratory sinus arrhythmia and parasympathetic cardiac control: some basic issues concerning quantification, application and implications. In: Grossman P, Janssen K, Vaitl D (eds), Cardiorespiratory and cardiosomatic psychophysiology. Plenum Press, New York, pp. 117-138.

20. Saul JP, Berger RD, Albrecht P, Stein SP, Chen MH, Cohen RJ (1991) Transfer function analysis of the circulation: unique insights into cardiovascular regulation. American Journal of Physiology 261:H1231-H1245

21. Porges SW (1995) Orienting in a defensive world: mammalian modifications of our evolutionary heritage. A Polyvagal Theory. Psychophysiology 32:301-318

22. Porges SW (1992) Vagal tone: Physiologic marker of stress vulnerability. Pediatrics 90:498-504

23. Valentinuzzi ME, Geddes LA (1974) The central component of the respiratory heart-rate response. Cardiovascular Research Center Bulletin 12:87-103

24. Akselrod S, Gordon D, Ubel FA, Shannon DC, Barger AC, Cohen RJ (1981) Power spectrum analysis of heart rate fluctuation: a quantitative probe of beat-to-beat cardiovascular control. Science 213:220-222

25. Pomeranz B, Macaulay RJB, Caudill MA, Kutz I, Adam D, Gordon D, Kilborn KA, Barger C, Shannon DC, Cohen RJ, Benson H. (1985) Assessment of autonomic function in humans by heart rate spectral analysis. American Journal of Physiology 248:H151 - H153

26. Bernardi L, Leuzzi S, Radaelli A, Passino C, Johnston JA, Sleight P (1994) Low frequency spontaneous fluctuations of R-R interval and blood pressure in conscious humans: a baroreceptor or central phenomenon? Clinical Science 87:647-654.

27. Vaschillo E, Lehrer P, Rishe N, Konstantinov M (submitted for publication) Frequency frequency characteristics of voluntarily-induced heart rhythm and blood pressure oscillations. UMDNJ–Robert Wood Johnson Medical School, Piscataway, NJ

28. Davidson S, Reina N, Shefi O, Hai-Tov U, Akselrod S (1997) Spectral analysis of heart rate fluctuations and optimum thermal management for low birth weight infants. Medical and Biological Engineering and Computing 35:619-625

29. Fleisher LA, Frank SM, Sessler DI, Cheng C, Matsukawa T, Vannier CA (1996) Thermoregulation and heart rate variability. Clinical Science 90:97-103.

30. Taylor JA, Carr DL, Meyers CW, Eckberg DL (1998) Mechanisms underlying very-low-frequency RR-interval oscillations in humans. Circulation 98:547-555

31. Vaschillo EG, Zingerman AM, Konstantinov MA, Menitsky DN (1983) Research on the resonance characteristics for cardiovascular system. Human Physiology 9:257-265.

32. Chernigovskaya NV, Vachillo EG, Petrash VV, Rusanovsky VV (1990) Voluntary regulation of the heart rate as a method of functional condition correction in neurotics. Human Physiology 16:58-64.

33. Vasilevskii NN, Sidorov IuA, Suvorov NB (1993) [Role of biorhythmologic processes in adaptation mechanisms and correction of regulatory dysfunctions] [Russian] Fiziologii Cheloveka 19:91-98.

34. Chernigovskaya NV, Vachillo EG, Rusanovsky BB, Kashkarova OE (1990) Instrumental autotraining of mechanisms for cardiovascular function regulation in treatment of neurotics [Russian]. The SS Korsakov's Journal of Neuropathology and Psychiatry 90:24-28.

35. Sidorov IuA, Vasilevskii (1994) [The physiological problems of biofeedback control by the heart rate]. [Russian] NNFiziol Zh Im I M Sechenova 80:1-7

36. Ogata M, Ikeda M., Kuratsune M (1984) Mortality among Japanese Zen priests. Journal of Epidemiology and Community Health 38:161-166

37. Lehrer PM, Sasaki Y, Saito Y (In press) Zazen and cardiac variability. Psychosomatic Medicine

38. Matsumoto H (1977) A psychological study of the relation between respiratory function and emotion. In: Akishige Y (ed) Psychological studies of Zen, Vol 1. Komazawa University, Tokyo, pp. 167-206.

Breathing Regulation in Zen Buddhism

Tadashi Chihara

Department of Psychology, Komazawa University, 1-23-1 Komazawa, Setagaya-ku, Tokyo 154-8525, Japan

Summary: Śākyamuni eventually denied Appāna-kajhāna (No-breathing Zen), a practice of hindering breathing, of inhaling and exhaling, through one's mouth and nose. He instead taught a special state for concentrating and giving deep attention to inhalation (āna) and exhalation (apāna) of breath, or Ānāpāna-sati, when calming and purifying one's mind, then entering meditation. There are six stages to Ānāpāna-sati, which T'ien-t'ai Chih-i (538-597) named "Lu Miao Fa Meng (the six entrances of enlightenment)". The sage classified breathing into four ways, of which he considered "Hsi" the correct one, concluding, "It is important for the regulation of breath to be natural." Zen master Dōgen (1200-1253) said inhalation and exhalation are neither long nor short. It is (the method of) the Greater Vehicle, but it is different from the Lesser Vehicle; it is not the Lesser Vehicle, but is different from the Greater Vehicle, he said. Rather, transcending such matter, he mentions his view with regards to "sloughing off body and mind naturally" and "No-thinking." Respiratory changes during *zazen* through breathing regulation indicate a lowered metabolism. The practice of *zazen* consists of three subjects: *Chō-shin* (regulation of the body); *Chō-soku* (regulation of breathing); and *Chō-jin* (regulation of the mind). These three subjects are very closely related to each other. "No-thinking" harmonizes the body, breathing and mind to form a harmonious whole, whereby we are able to contemplate the real existence of changeful things. Such is the significance of Ānāpāna-sati.

Key words: Ānāpāna-sati, T'ien-T'ai, Breathing regulation, *Zazen*, Innate breathing

The ancient Indians perceived that breathing was the most profound matter concerning the origin of the universe, as presented in the Ṛg-Veda [1] and the Upaniṣad [2]. Prāṇa maintains the internal life of individuals, as well as being recognized as both the subjective and supreme principle of the universe. Furthermore, in the Yoga–sūtra [3], a fundamental sacred book of the Yoga school, the suspension of breathing is classified into four types [4], and regulation of breathing has a significant meaning as a readiness stage prior to deepening one's meditation.

ŚĀKYAMUNI'S ĀNĀPĀNA-SATI

Buddhism was greatly influenced by the practice of Yoga. After six years mortification, Śākyamuni eventually denied Appāna-kajhāna (No-breathing Zen), which hinders the inhaling and exhaling through one's mouth and nose. Śākyamuni instead taught a special state to concentrate and pay deep attention to inhalation (āna) and exhalation (apāna), called Ānāpāna-sati, before calming and purifying one's mind, then entering meditation. Āna means "breathing in", while Apana means "breathing out". Sati is to concentrate. When the practice is applied properly, breathing is controlled and the mind is calmed. And thus Ānāpāna-sati is often called *Susokukan* (meditation by counting one's breath).

The Chapter of Ānāpāna in Vol. VII of the Ekottaragama-sūtra [5] describes Ānāpāna-sati as "connecting your mind with nose, realizing of long breath when making a long exhalation, realizing long breath when taking a long inhalation, also knowing short breath when taking a short exhalation, also knowing short breath when taking a short inhalation..." The Chapter of Kōen in Vol. II of Ekottaragama-sūtra [6] adds, "you should perceive that a long breath when breathing long, and a short breath when breathing short, breath becomes long or short when taking long or short breathing." According to these chapters, the very practice of Ānāpāna-sati is to contemplate an inhalation / exhalation and long / short respiration by keeping one's body and mind calm. The primary point of Ānāpāna-sati is to understand long and short breathing. The discipline consists of two basic patterns; prolonged exhalation – prolonged inhalation; and shortened exhalation – shortened inhalation. The basic two patterns are further divided into four categories [7] and are linked with four types of meditation (Shi-nenjo) [8], which eliminate all false views besides the fundamentals of the practice in Buddhism. Finally, the two basic patterns were subdivided into 16 methods (solasa-vatthūni) [9].

There are six stages to Ānāpāna-sati, which are as follows:

i) *Su* (gaṇanā): to count one's breaths while meditating to prevent distraction, of which there are many manuals for counting.

ii) *Zui* (anugama): to breath naturally while meditating.

iii) *Shi* (sthāna): to stop discriminatory thinking due to Appanā.

iv) *Kan* (upalakṣaṇa): to contemplate a specific subject clearly.

v) *Gen* or *Ten* (vivartanā): to perceive one's own mind as being unreal.

vi) *Jo* (pariśuddhi): to realize that there is no basis for illusion.

T'ien-t'ai Chih-i (538-597) named these six stages the "Lu Miao Fa Meng (the six entrances to enlightenment)," for he considered the six stages were linked to entering Nirvāṇa. In the Vimutti-magga [10], however, the practice consists of four ways; *San, Zuichiku, Anchi and Zuigan*. Meanwhile the Visuddhi-magga [11] has eight ways, whereby the Phusanā and Tesaṁ Patipassanā are added to T'ien-t'ai's six stages. The objective of Ānāpāna-sati, essentially, was to let one's body and mind be calm when entering Zen-meditation. Beyond that, its theory was mad so complicated as to confuse most practitioners. In later days, Zen sects have abbreviated such intricate rules concerning *Susoku*.

CALMING AND DISCERNMENT IN T'IEN-T'AI

The T'ien-T'ai Hsiao Chih-Kuan [12], on whose teachings a number of Zen-meditation manuals are based, states the significance of harmonizing five things; food, sleep, body, breathing and mind. He also mentions four types of breathing, summarized as follows:

i) Feng (audible):When one sits in meditation, if the breath is perceptible to the ear, it is audible.

ii) Ch'uan (gasping): Although the breath is not audible, it is gasping if it is not free and is obstructing.

iii) Ch'i (coarse): Although the breath is not heard and is free, it is coarse if it is not fine.

iv) Hsi (restful): When the breath is neither audible nor obstructed nor coarse, but is continuous, being barely perceptible and so fine that it is almost imperceptible, with the resultant comfort and easiness, it is restful.

T'ien-T'ai says "Hsi" is the right way of breathing. In addition, he gives the following practical instruction for regulating breathing.

i) Calm the mind by concentrating the breathing below the abdomen.

ii) Relax the body and mind.
iii) Visualize breathing coming in and going out through all pores freely and unobstructedly.

The healing chapter in Vol. IX of the Hsiao Chih-Kuan refers to six types of breathing; i) puffing, ii) expelling, iii) shouting, iv) sighing, v) soothing and vi) restful.
Moreover, it shows twelve types of breathing method and teaches the way of curing diseases by means of "contemplation" [13].
Finally, T'ien-T'ai states, "if the breath is neither obstructed nor imperceptible, it is the regulation of breath," and concludes "it is important for the regulation of breath to be natural."

ZEN MASTER DŌGEN'S BREATHING REGULATION

Zen master Dōgen (1200-1253), who founded the Sōtō sect, wrote and defined the techniques and manners of Zen-meditation in *Fukan zazen gi*. In *Bendōhō* [14] treatise he says to regulate breathing is to "breathe quietly through our nostrils, not hard or noisy, not too long or too short, too slow or too fast." Additionally, in Vol. V of *Eiheikōroku* [15], he outlines his view on breathing regulation as follows:

...."The followers of Lesser Vehicle (Hīnayāna) use the counting of breath to control the breathing, but the pursuit of the way of the Buddha and Patriarchs is very different from that of the Lesser Vehicle The Greater Vehicle (Mahāyāna) also has a method for regulating the breath: it is to know [when the breath is long] that this is a long breath, and to know [when it is short] that this is a short breath."...

My former master, T'ien-t'um, has said, ..."the breath enters the field of the abdomen (cinnabar), but it does not come from anywhere; hence, it is neither long nor short. The breath exists from the field of the abdomen, but it does not go anywhere; hence, it is neither short nor long"...

"I (Dōgen) would simply say that it is [the method of] the Greater Vehicle, but it is different from the Lesser Vehicle; it is not the Lesser Vehicle, but it is different from the Greater Vehicle. I would say that inhalation and exhalation are neither long nor short."

Pai-chang said, "the Essence of my law is beyond and in the Greater and Lesser Vehicles, and it is not different from the Greater and Lesser Vehicles. You should act on the norm between the Greater and Lesser Vehicles"...

Dōgen would say otherwise: "I act beyond the limitation of the differences in these Vehicles. I transcend the Greater and Lesser Vehicles themselves, and do not stay in the middle of them."...

For Dōgen, breathing regulation in the Greater and Lesser Vehicles, and the difference between long breath and short breath are no longer problems. Transcending such matter, he instead mentions his view with regard to "sloughing off body and mind naturally," and "No-thinking."

Zen master Keizan (1267-1325), the so-called "second founder" of the Sōtō sect, in *Zazen yōjin ki* [16] said the following concerning breathing regulation:

"Keep breathing long if you have a long breath, keep breathing short if you have a short breath, you should stay in a natural state anyway. When gradually regulating your breath, and then, forming a harmonious whole in a breath in accordance with relaxed inhalation and exhalation, your body and mind are stabilized by themselves. Thereafter, you do continuous respiration through nostrils naturally."

RESPIRATORY CHANGE DURING *ZAZEN*

What then are the respiratory physiological effects when meditating in *zazen* without any tensions, rage or an evil mind?

According to Akishige, respiration during breathing regulation of *zazen* is characterized as follows (Akishige, 1975) [17]:

i) Slight, abdominal breathing. Movement of the diaphragm is increased, abdominal cavity pressure rises to a high level.

ii) Expiration time is longer than inspiration time, and when the frequency of respiration is reduced, expiration is made into a tension phase, while inspiration is made into a relaxation phase.

iii) Ventilation volume is lowered, and a decrease is noted in oxygen (O_2) consumption and carbon dioxide (CO_2) production.

iv) There is an increase in ventilation volume per cycle of respiration (tidal volume), and an increase in the elimination of carbon dioxide per one cycle of respiration.

v) Respiratory quotient (CO_2/O_2) is stabilized and lower than normal volume.

vi) There is a slight decrease in the partial pressure of carbon dioxide ($PaCO_2$) in expired air.

vii) The pH of blood and urine turns normal acidosis.

These physiological changes during *zazen* indicate a lowered metabolism. Oxygen consumption of an experienced *zazen* practitioner is on an extremely low level. This, it is believed, is due mainly to reduced oxygen consumption in the brain.

As mentioned above, *zazen* respiration results from abdominal inspiration and expiration with short inhalation and long inhalation, so that the volume of energy consumption is reduced. However, even though less-experienced practitioners try to count breath and to control their postures, desirable results would not be obtained as Zen priests do. The practice of *zazen* consists of three subjects: *Chō-shin* (body-regulation); *Chō-soku* (breathing-regulation); and *Chō-jin* (mind regulation). These subjects are very closely related to each other. The three parts are contained in the whole, the whole (one) is in the three parts. Whichever *Chō-shin, Chō-soku* and *Chō-jin* are realized, the other two subjects are essential.

INNATE BREATHING

Breathing enables one to unite body and mind with the outer world; the universe; as well as being a "bridge" between body and mind. Devoting discipline to inhalation and exhalation (i.e. *zazen*) in everyday life is "No-thinking" which harmonizes body, breathing and mind, them forms a harmonious whole. Thereby, we are able to contemplate the real existence of changeful things. Here lies the significance of Ānāpāna-sati [18].

In ordinary life where we feel full of stresses, the so-called "natural breathing" we do unconsciously and reflectively is a wrong "distorted breathing". Breathing regulation enables one to harmonize body with mind, and to explore our true life and real existence through consciously controlling breath, choosing to concentrate on it, and in so recovering "innate breathing" of our own. Realizing this unconscious innate breathing, though, is quite difficult. Breathing regulation is done by means of intentional control. It must nonetheless be done unconsciously and automatically. We cannot accomplish such regulation as a daily activity until the innate breath becomes ordinal. Devoting discipline to inhalation and exhalation (*zazen*) in everyday life means

"No-thinking" that is the harmonization of the body, breath and mind, in other words, the formation of a harmonious whole in breath.

REFERENCES

1. Wilson H.H. (1977) Ṛg-Veda Saṃhita, Text in Nagari, english translation, notes and appendices, etc. Enlarged and arranged by Nag Sharan, Delhi, Nag Publishers, 6 volumes.

2. Deussen P. (1980) Sixty Upanisads of the Veda, Translated from German by Bedekar, V.M. and Palsule, G.B., 2parts, Delhi, etc, Motilal Banarsidass.

3. Meisig K. (1988) Yogasūtra-konkordanz. Wiesbaden: Otto Horrassowitz. pp 49-56.
   Woods J.H. (1914) The Yoga-system of patañjali, or the ancient hindu doctrine of concentrations of mind. Embracing the mnemonic rules, called Yoga-sūtras, of patañjali and the comment, called Yoga-Bhāshya, attributed to Veda-vyāsa and the explanation, called Tattvavaiçāradī, of vāchaspati-Miçra, trans. from the original Sanskrit, Harvard oriental series, 17, Harvard University press, 2nd ed (1927). Cambridge, Mass.

4. Yoga-sūtra, II, 49-53.

5. Taishō shinshū daizōkyō, [Taishō Tripitaka (T.T.)] vol.2, 581.

6. Ibid., T.T.,2:556.

7. Ibid., T.T.,2:556.a-b.

8. The four insights. The insights that the body is impure (1. Shin-nenjo), perception leads to suffering (2.Ju-nenjo), the mind is impermanent (3.Shi-nenjo), and the world is transient (4.Hō-nenjo). The four stations or bases of mindfulness are included in the 37 elements of enlightenment (sanjūshichi dōbon).

9. Vinayapiṭaka, Ed., P.T.S. III, pp 70-71. Majjhima-Nikāya, I, p.21, III, p.2, p.9. Saṃyutta-Nikaya V, pp 1-329, p.40. Anguttara-Nikaya, V, p.109. Zō-agon-gyō 803 Saṃyuktāgama, T.T.2, 206-a-b. Makasōgi-ritsu Mahāsaṃghika, T.T.22: 254c-255a. Jūju-ritsu sarvāstivādin-Vinaya, T.T.23: 8a-b.

10. T.T.32: 429.

11. Viuddhi-magga, Ed., P.T.S. pp 6-293.

12. Lu K'uan Yü, (1969) The secrets of Chinese meditation, Samuel weiser,inc. York Beach, maine, pp 9-162.
    Sekiguchi Shindai(1991) Gendaigo yaku Tendai shō shikan. Tokyo:Daitō shuppan, pp 39-46.

13. Lu K'uan Yü. Ibid, p.149. Sekiguchi, Ibid, pp116-117.

14. Ōkubo Dōshū Ed., (1970) Dōgen zenji zenshū, vol.2, Tokyo: Chikuma Shobō, pp 313-319.
    Carl Bielefeldt(1988) Dōgens Manuals of Zen meditation. U.C. press: Berkeley.

15. Eiheikōroku; Ibid, Dōgen zenji zenshū, vol.2, pp 7-200.
    Terada Tōru (1995) Dōgen oshō kōroku, vol.1, pp 373-376.

The Eihei-kōroku trans by Yokoi Yūhō, (1987) Sankibō Buddhist Book-store, Tokyo, pp 178-180.

16. T.T. 82: Zazen yōjinki, by Keizan, sōtō shū zensho, (1929-38), Shūgen : vol.2 : pp 423-427.

17. Akishige Yoshiharu (1975) Zen no shinrigaku, kōza Bukkyō shisō, vol. 4 Risōsha, Tokyo.
Akishige Yoshiharu (Ed, 1977) Psychological studies on Zen, II, Bulletin of the Zen Institute of Komazawa University, 1, pp 1-63.

18. T.T., 15: 163c. Bussetsu Dai anpan shuikyō.
Ui Hakuju (1971) An seikō, Dokkyōshi kenkyū, Iwanami shoten, Tokyo, pp 201-244.

Respiration and Emotion (II)

GAINING INSIGHT INTO THE FACTORS THAT INFLUENCE THE VARIABILTY OF BREATHING

Thomas Brack, MD and Martin J. Tobin, MD
Division of Pulmonary and Critical Care Medicine, Edward Hines Jr. VA Hospital, Mailing
Route 111N, Hines IL 60141, USA

Summary: Remarkably little is known about the mechanisms that regulate the pattern of breathing, and most research on the control of breathing has been confined to measuring mean responses of the respiratory controller to physiological perturbations. We analyzed variability of breathing in healthy subjects under different conditions by partitioning variational activity in a random and a non-random (correlated and oscillatory) fraction. For volume components, hyperoxic hypercapnia decreased the relative contribution of random variability and increased the non-random behavior; it also increased the number of consecutive breath lags displaying significant autocorrelation coefficients ("short-term memory"). The increases in correlated behavior and "short-term memory" during hyperoxic hypercapnia may have been the consequence of carbon dioxide-mediated increases in afterdischarge of the respiratory controller. Elastic loading increased the random fraction of variational activity in inspiratory time whereas it decreased the random variability of tidal volume. As a means of minimizing dyspnea when compensating for an inspiratory load, the advantage of prolonging inspiratory time as opposed to increasing the magnitude of inspiratory muscle effort may explain the opposing changes in the random fractions of tidal volume and inspiratory time. A resistive load of 3 cm $H_2O/L/sec$ decreased the random variability of breath components, whereas a load of 6 cm $H_2O/L/sec$ increased random variability compared to both rest and the smaller load. The proximity of the smaller resistive load to the perception threshold can explain this apparent paradox. In conclusion, we have shown that hyperoxic hypercapnia, elastic loading, and resistive loading cause specific and unique changes in different fractions of variational activity; the insight gained from analysis of respiratory variability advances our understanding of the control of breathing.

Key words: variability of breathing; hyperoxic hypercapnia; elastic load; resistive load

INTRODUCTION

Most research into the respiratory control system has focused on mean values of variables reflecting respiratory motor output. In contrast, little or no attention has been paid to the breath-to-breath variability of respiratory output. The description of physiological processes by mean values can provide only a blurred silhouette of reality. A sharper contour is provided by quantifying the variability of a parameter around the mean. Analysis of breath variability can expand our understanding of physiological mechanisms involved in the control of breathing (1). It may also serve as a marker of disease severity and prognosis. For example, a decrease in heart rate variability predicts increased mortality after myocardial (2, 3).

130

The problem that arises from an analysis based on the calculation of the mean response of the respiratory control system to a perturbation is illustrated in Figure 1. The mean of the total minute ventilation in the lower panel is identical to that in the upper panel. Since most published literature on control of breathing in humans is based on the mean response to a perturbation, these two responses would be considered the same. Yet, simple inspection of the two patterns indicates that the behavior of the respiratory control system is very different in the two instances. With sophisticated signal analysis techniques, it is possible to partition the deviations of the magnitude of a breath component from its mean into a non-random (correlated/oscillatory) fraction and a random, white noise [w(n)] fraction (4-9) (Figure 2). In healthy volunteers, we have shown that physiologic perturbations, such as hyperoxic hypercapnia (8), elastic loading (7), and resistive loading (9), cause unique changes in the different fractions of variational activity -- findings that enhance our understanding of respiratory regulation.

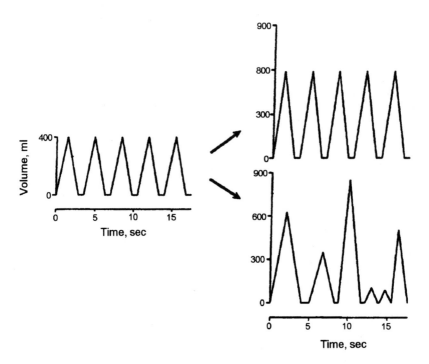

Fig. 1: *Left:* Normal pattern of breathing with a tidal volume of 400 ml and respiratory frequency of 17 breaths per minute. *Right:* An increase in ventilatory demands is met by an increase in minute ventilation to 10 L/min (from 7 L/min). In the upper panel, this is achieved solely by an increase in tidal volume with no change in respiratory timing. The total minute ventilation in the lower panel is identical to that in the upper panel, although the behavior of the respiratory control system is clearly very different. (From Tobin MJ (ed). Principles and Practice of Intensive Care Monitoring: p.488. McGraw-Hill, Inc. New York, 1998,; with permission)

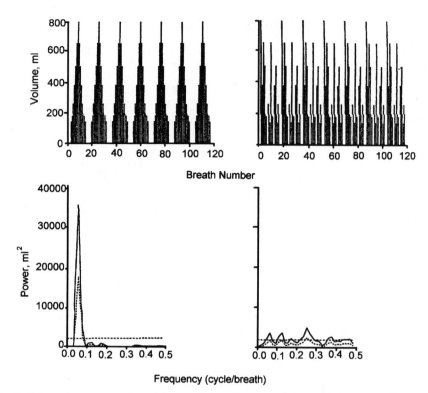

Fig. 2: Schematic representation of the superiority of autocorrelation analysis over coefficients of variation in assessment of variability of breathing. The mean $\pm$ SD for tidal volume are the same for the two time series, 296 $\pm$ 246 ml, and, thus, the coefficients of variation are identical. However, simple inspection indicates that the time series of the *left* exhibits obvious periodicity, while that on the *right* has an erratic pattern. Fast Fourier transformation reveals a significant peak in the *left-hand* data set, in contrast to the broad frequency band distribution for the *right-hand* data set. On fractionation, uncorrelated random (white noise) behavior accounts for 99.9% of the variational activity on the *right*, but only 10% of that on the *left*.

HYPEROXIC HYPERCAPNIA

Although an enormous literature pertains to the influence of hypercapnia on mean changes in respiratory output, research on the effect of carbon dioxide on the variability of breathing in humans is scant to non-existent. To investigate the role of central chemoreceptor stimulation on variational activity of breathing, we recorded ventilation non-obtrusively in 14 healthy subjects before and during steady-state hyperoxic hypercapnia **(8)**. Hyperoxia diminishes activity of the peripheral chemoreceptors, such that step changes in carbon dioxide tension are considered to represent a relatively pure central chemoreceptor stimulus **(10, 11)**. Compared with air, an increase in end-tidal carbon dioxide of as approximately 13 torr significantly increased the total variance of minute ventilation and tidal volume, and decreased that of inspiratory time and expiratory time. Hyperoxic hypercapnia increased the autocorrelation coefficient at a lag of 1 breath for minute ventilation (from 0.194 to 0.329, $p < 0.05$), and the number of consecutive breath lags having significant autocorrelation coefficients for minute ventilation (from 2.7 to 22.5, $p < 0.01$) and tidal volume (from 3.2 to 15.1, $p < 0.01$) **(Figure 3).**

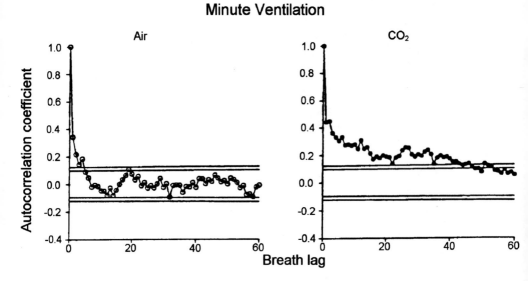

Fig. 3: Autocorrelogram of minute ventilation in a subject during air and hyperoxic hypercapnia (CO_2). The autocorrelation coefficient at a lag of 1 breath increased from 0.34 during air breathing to 0.44 during hyperoxic hypercapnia. The number of breath lags with significant serial correlations ($p < 0.01$) increased from 4 during air breathing to 49 during hyperoxic hypercapnia. On the autocorrelograms, points lying outside the inner pair of isopleths are statistically different than zero, at $p < 0.05$, and outside the outer pair of isopleths, at $p < 0.01$ **(8)**.

The mechanism underlying the dependence of breath components on the characteristics of the preceding respiratory cycle is unknown. That minute ventilation increased by 3-fold suggests that afterdischarge (facilitatory memory) may also have been activated **(12, 13)** -- perhaps, by a direct effect of hypercapnia **(14)**. An additional contributor to the increase in correlated behavior may have been removal of the rapid and fine-adjustment actions of the peripheral chemoreceptors as a result of hyperoxia **(10)**. Thus, deviations of minute ventilation will return more slowly to the mean level.

Spectral analysis revealed that the frequency of significant oscillations in minute ventilation decreased from 0.12 to 0.04 cycle/breath, signifying an increase in the number of breaths per cycle from 8 to 25. Assuming an average breath duration of 3.5 sec **(15)**, this is equivalent to an increase in cycle time from approximately 28 to 88 sec. This cycle length is compatible with the time constant of the central chemoreceptors, approximately 75 sec **(16)**, suggesting that activation of central chemoreceptors played an important role in the development of the low-frequency oscillations.

Fractionation of the variational activity revealed that hyperoxic hypercapnia decreased the uncorrelated random [w(n)] fraction of minute ventilation (from 91.5 to 76.7%, p = 0.05) and tended to increase its correlated fraction (from 8.6 to 20.1%, p = 0.06). The autocorrelation coefficient at a lag of 1 breath for minute ventilation during hyperoxic hypercapnia was negatively correlated with a quasi-steady-state measurement of carbon dioxide gain, suggesting that the higher the carbon dioxide gain, the more "noisy" the breath-to-breath variability in minute ventilation during hyperoxic hypercapnia.

In summary, although the increased variability of minute ventilation and tidal volume with hyperoxic hypercapnia was predominantly due to uncorrelated random fluctuations, a significant portion resulted from increased correlated behavior accompanied by the development of low-frequency oscillations with a cycle time consistent with central chemoreceptor activation.

ELASTIC LOADING

Patients with a pathologically increased intrinsic elastic load, such as those with restrictive lung disease, have a rapid shallow breathing pattern. To simulate this abnormal state, numerous studies have been performed using external elastic loading. Virtually all of these studies have been confined to assessing the mean response and little is known about changes of respiratory variability during elastic loading. Elastic loading forces the respiratory controller to compensate through an increase in motor output while also minimizing dyspnea that can result from increased output (17). These potentially conflicting challenges may limit the freedom of the controller to vary breath components.

To investigate the possibility that an elastic load decreases respiratory variability, we studied 11 healthy subjects breathing at rest and with inspiratory elastic loads of 9 and 18 cm H_2O/L (i.e., double and triple normal elastance) for 1 hr each (7). Compared with rest, a load of 18 cm H_2O/L decreased the total variance of tidal volume and expiratory time (p < 0.01 in both instances), and increased the total variance of inspiratory time (p < 0.03).

Fractionation of the total variance revealed that these alterations were due to changes in w(n) behavior, while the correlated and oscillatory fractions were not significantly affected (Figure 4). That the random fractions of the variability of the two inspiratory breath components, tidal volume and inspiratory time, moved in opposite directions was, at first glance, surprising; however, this probably reflects compensatory strategies of the respiratory controller to avoid deterioration in gas exchange when challenged with an elastic load, while also avoiding dyspnea (17, 18).

Preservation of minute ventilation, as observed in our subjects, can be achieved by either an increase in driving pressure or by prolongation of inspiratory time, both of which occurred. To avoid discomfort, the controller can choose to strictly minimize the increase in driving pressure and prolong inspiratory time, since this strategy restores tidal volume with less distortion of the length-tension relationship of the inspiratory muscles (18, 19). The observed increase in random variability of inspiratory time and decrease in random variability of tidal volume indicate, indirectly, a decrease in the variability of driving pressure. As a means of minimizing dyspnea when compensating for an inspiratory load, the advantage of prolonging inspiratory time as opposed to increasing driving pressure may explain the opposing changes in the random fractions of tidal volume and inspiratory time.

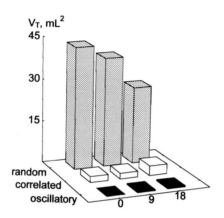

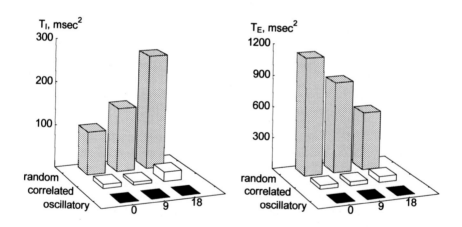

Fig. 4: Total variance (top of each column) of tidal volume (V_T), inspiratory time (T_I) and expiratory time (T_E) in 11 healthy subjects during resting breathing (load 0) and while breathing against inspiratory elastic load of 9 and 18 cm H_2O/L per second. The latter load decreased the variance of V_T and T_E, while it increased that of T_I. Partitioning of the variational activity into correlated, oscillatory, and random fractions revealed that the alterations were due to changes in the random (white noise) fraction of the breath components; the correlated and oscillatory fractions did not change significantly (7).

RESISTIVE LOADING

Investigation of the response to external resistive loads has yielded important insights into the function of the respiratory control system (17), but, again, most research has focused on the mean responses. In 18 healthy subjects, we found that inspiratory resistive loading altered variational activity according to the size of the load (Figure 5). A load of 3 cm $H_2O/L/sec$ decreased the total variance of minute ventilation and expiratory time secondary to decreases in the random fractions; this load also increased the autocorrelation coefficient at a lag of 1 breath for tidal volume (from 0.17 to 0.24, $p < 0.05$). A load of 6 cm $H_2O/L/sec$ increased the total and random fractions of variational activity of inspiratory time and the correlated fraction of tidal volume; this load also decreased the autocorrelation coefficient at a lag of 1 breath for minute ventilation (from 0.13 to 0.09, $p < 0.05$). Compared with a resistive load of 3 cm H_2O/sec, the load of 6 cm $H_2O/L/sec$ increased the total and random fractions of variational activity of all breath components (9).

The proximity of the smaller resistive load to the perception threshold (20, 21) can explain the apparent paradox that the smaller load decreased the total and random variational activity of breath components, whereas the higher load increased the total and random variability compared to both rest and the smaller load. Respiratory control during wakefulness is accepted as being conjointly influenced by automatic and behavioral factors (22, 23). Overall respiratory motor output is determined by an automatic control system in the brainstem, and behavioral influences from supramedullary structures (23); the former system is dominant during Stage III/IV non rapid eye movement (NREM) sleep, while behavioral factors can override it in the conscious state -- the so called "wakefulness drive to breathe" (24). A load below or around the perception threshold would be expected to emphasize automatic regulation and to decrease random variability, while eventually increasing correlated variability. A suprathreshold load necessarily activates behavioral (cortical) control, and by prevailing over automatic regulation, may have been responsible for the increased random variability of breath components with a load of 6 cm $H_2O/L/sec$.

These observations suggest that the fractions of variational activity have different physiological implications: unstructured random variability may be a measure of behavioral influences, whereas the structured correlated fraction may represent automatic influence on respiratory control.

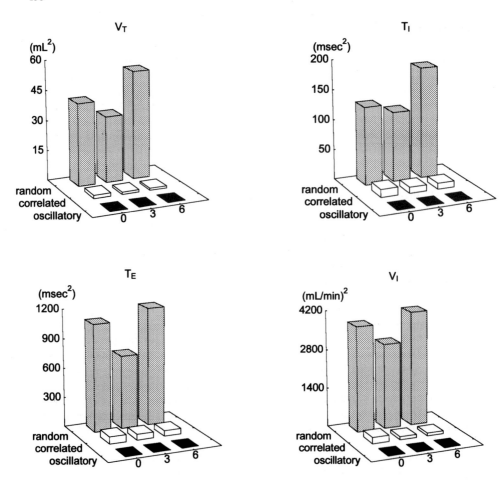

Fig. 5: Partitioning of total variances of tidal volume (V_T), inspiratory time (T_I), expiratory time (T_E) and minute ventilation ($\dot{V}_I$) into fractions of oscillatory (black columns), correlated (white columns), and uncorrelated random (stippled columns) behavior during resting breathing (0 cm $H_2O/L/sec$) and with resistive loads of 3 and 6 cm $H_2O/L/sec$. Compared with rest, the load of 6 cm $H_2O/L/sec$ increased the random fraction of T_I ($p < 0.01$) and the correlated fraction of V_T ($p < 0.05$). Compared with resting breathing, the load of 3 cm $H_2O/L/sec$ decreased the random fractions of $\dot{V}_I$ ($p < 0.05$ in both instances). Compared with a load of 3 cm $H_2O/L/sec$, the load of 6 cm $H_2O/L/sec$ increased the random fractions of V_T, T_I and $\dot{V}_I$ ($p < 0.01$ in all 3 instances) and T_E ($p < 0.05$) **(9)**.

CONCLUSION

Analysis of the gross variability and its subsequent partitioning into random and non-random fractions makes it possible to describe the breathing pattern more precisely than in previous investigations which focused on the mean respiratory output. The new and expanded knowledge of respiratory variability can lead to a better physiologic understanding of factors that can influence control of breathing under different conditions. Increases in non-random variability and "short-term memory" during hyperoxic hypercapnia may indicate a specific chemical response (afterdischarge) of the respiratory controller. The increase of the random fraction of inspiratory time along with the simultaneous decrease of random variability of tidal volume during elastic loading may reflect the controller's attempt to compensate for the load while simultaneously minimizing dyspnea. Finally, the importance of the perception threshold and the cortical influence on the breathing pattern can be elucidated through changes in variability during resistive loading. These examples illustrate the potential of analyzing respiratory variability for rendering greater insight into the performance of the respiratory controller. As such, the application of signal analysis techniques holds considerable promise as a means of advancing our understanding of respiratory diseases and their pathophysiology.

REFERENCES

1. Bruce, E.N. and J.A. Daubenspeck. Mechanisms and analysis of ventilatory stability. In J.A. Dempsey and A.I. Pack, editors; Regulation of Breathing, 2nd ed. Marcel Dekker, Inc., New York. 1995: 285-313.
2. Bigger, J.T., Jr, J.L. Fleiss, R.C. Steinman, L.M. Rolnitzky, R.E. Kleiger, and J.N. Rottman. 1992. Frequency domain measures of heart period variability and mortality after myocardial infarction. Circulation. 85:164-171.
3. Kleiger, R.E., J.P. Miller, J.T. Bigger, Jr., and A.J. Moss. 1987. Decreased heart rate variability and its association with increased mortality after acute myocardial infarction. Am. J. Cardiol. 59:256-262.
4. Modarreszadeh M, Bruce EN, Gothe B. Non random variability in respiratory cycle parameters of humans during stage 2 sleep. J Appl Physiol 1990;69:630-639.
5. Tobin MJ, Perez W, Guenther SM et al. The pattern of breathing during successful and unsuccessful trials of weaning from mechanical ventilation. Am Rev Respir Dis 1986;134:1111-1118.
6. Tobin MJ, Yang KL, Jubran A, Lodato RF. Interrelationship of breath components in neighboring breaths of normal eupneic subjects. Am J Respir Crit Care Med 1995;152:1967-76.
7. Brack T, Jubran A, Tobin MJ. Effect of elastic loading on variational activity of breathing. Am J Respir Crit Care Med 1997;155:1341-1348.
8. Jubran A, Grant BJB, Tobin MJ. Effect of hyperoxic hypercapnia on variational activity of breathing. Am J Respir Crit Care Med 1997;156:1129-1139.
9. Brack T, Jubran A, Tobin MJ. Effect of resistive loading on variational activity of breathing. Am J Respir Crit Care Med 1998; 157:1756-1763.

10. Gardner WN. The pattern of breathing following step changes of alveolar partial pressures of carbon dioxide and oxygen in man. J Physiol (London) 1980;300:55-73.

11. Ledlie JF, Kelsen SG, Cherniack NS, Fishman AP. Effects of hypercapnia and hypoxia on phrenic nerve activity and respiratory timing. J Appl Physiol 1981;51:732-738.

12. Badr MS, Skatrud J, Dempsey JA. Determinants of post-stimulus potentiation in humans during NREM sleep. J Appl Physiol 1992;73:1958-1871.

13. Ahmed M, Giesbrecht GG, Serrette C, Georgopoulos D, Anthonisen NR. Respiratory short-term potentiation (after-discharge) in elderly humans. Respir Physiol 1993;93:165-173.

14. Engwall MJA, Smith CA, Dempsey JA, Bisgard GE. Ventilatory afterdischarge and central respiratory drive interactions in the awake goat. J Appl Physiol 1994;76:416-423.

15. Tobin MJ, Mador MJ, Guenther SM, et al. Variability of resting respiratory center drive and timing in healthy subjects. J Appl Physiol 1988; 65:309-317.

16. Swanson GD, Bellville JW. Step changes in end-tidal CO_2: methods and implications. J Appl Physiol 1975;39:377-385.

17. Younes M. Mechanisms of respiratory load compensation. Dempsey JA, Pack AI (eds). Regulation of breathing. 2nd ed. Marcel Dekker, Inc. New York, 1995, p 867-922.

18. Campbell EJM, Howell JBL. The sensation of breathlessness. Br Med Bull 1963;19:36-40.

19. Younes M, Riddle W. Relation between respiratory neural output and tidal volume. J Appl Physiol 1984;56:1110-1119.

20. Daubenspeck JA, Rhodes ES. Effect of perception of mechanical loading on human respiratory pattern regulation. J Appl Physiol 1995;79:83-93.

21. Zechman FW, Wiley RL. Afferent inputs to breathing: respiratory sensation. In: Cherniack NS, Widdicombe JG, eds. Handbook of Physiology. The Respiratory System. Control of Breathing, Bethesda, MD: American Physiological Society, Sec 3, Vol 2, part 1:449-474.

22. Guz A. Brain, breathing and breathlessness. Respir Physiol 1997;109:197-204.

23. von Euler C. Brainstem mechanisms for generation and control of breathing pattern. In: Cherniack NS, Widdicombe JG (eds). Handbook of physiology: the respiratory system. Control of Breathing. Bethesda, Am Physiol Soc, 1986, p1-67.

24. Fink BR. Influence of cerebral activity in wakefulness on regulation of breathing. J Appl Physiol 1961;16:15-20.

Facilitation and Inhibition of Breathing During Changes in Emotion

Akio Umezawa

Department of Psychology, Fukui University, 3-9-1 Bunkyo, Fukui 910-8507, Japan

Summary: This article dealt with some issues concerning about links between respiration and emotion. Firstly, our recent studies on stress and respiration suggested that the central respiratory drive mechanism changes sensitively to psychological stressors, and also that the central timing mechanism and gas exchange system maintain stable during stress. Secondly, respiratory changes under detection of deception, which is thought to be stressful situation for a subject, are characterized by inhibitory breathing. Thirdly, these results obtained in several experiments suggested that some emotional experiences cause facilitation of breathing and that other emotional experience cause inhibitory breathing. Additional research is necessary to clarify which feeling induces facilitation of breathing and which feeling induces inhibitory breathing.

Key words: respiration, emotion, stress, respiratory central mechanism, inhibitory breathing, gas exchange

Breathing control as a relaxation strategy

In Japan, there is an empirical knowledge that control of breathing is an effective strategy to calm down during stressful situations in the daily life. In our country, there are many traditional expressions used a term of 'breath'. We say breath is '*iki*' in Japanese. There are almost seventy expressions used '*iki*', for example, '*Iki o totonoeru*' in Japanese, that is 'making breathe stable' in English. This expression means 'calming down'. We can observe that Japanese people have these empirical knowledge regardless of age. In my previous study [1], two hundred and forty-one male and female undergraduates completed the questionnaire concerning stressful events in the real life and relaxation strategies they used to overcome these stressful events. Fig. 1 shows the result of one question about relaxation strategies: 'How you control yourself under the stressful situation in your daily life'. The result clearly shows that the most numerous relaxation strategy is *deep breathing*. About 60 percents of subjects reported that they control breathing to calm down in their stressful situation. Many subjects answer this question that diaphragmatic breathing is an effective strategy to calm down. The result suggests that breathing control is the most popular relaxation strategy in our country.

Breathing patterns are considered to be closely related to consciousness in Japan. In experiences such as the silent meditation of "zen", great importance is placed especially upon breathing exercise and there are those who are concerned about its mental and somatic influences. The foresighted study conducted by Hitoshi Ishikawa [2] found that predominantly abdominal-diaphragmatic breathing is effective in the treatment of essential hypertension. In relaxation therapy in Western medicine, for example, Bensonian relaxation [3], subjects focus attention on their breathing and repeat the one word silently with each breath. Our empirical knowledge and clinical observation show that breathing control is an effective relaxation strategy. However there have been few basic studies which supports these empirical and clinical observations and which clarify the relationship between relaxation and respiratory functions. There have been also few studies confirmed that breathing control facilitates the depth of psychophysiological relaxation. Our empirical knowledge is not yet scientifically established. In this article we will discuss on the relationship between emotional experience and respiration. Our recent experiments concerning about emotion and respiration showed that hyperventilation

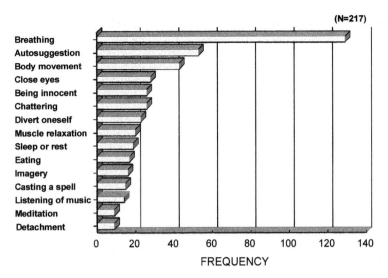

Fig. 1. Relaxation Strategies reported by 217 Japanese undergraduates subjects to the following question: "How you control yourself under the stressful situations in your daily life.

emerges in some emotional state and that hypoventilation emerges in other emotional state. In this article, I will discuss which psychological factors influence respiratory facilitation or inhibition

Effects of stress on breathing pattern and ventilation

Wientjes, Grossman, & Gaillard [4] stated that rate and depth of respiration, which have been traditional respiratory parameters in the psychophysiological studies, do not exhibit constant changes to various laboratory stressors such as mental arithmetic, a stress film, cold pressor, and reaction time task to avoid electronic shocks, and so on. Respiration rate may increase or decrease and tidal volume may increase or decrease, or remained unaltered under different behavioral

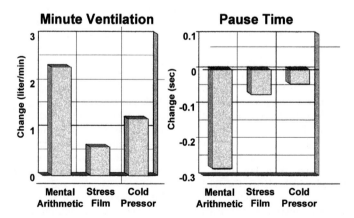

Fig. 2. Changes in minute ventilation (left) and post expiratory pause time (right) during mental arithmetic, a stress film, and cold pressor.

conditions. In my previous study [5, 6], twenty male subjects participated in all three sessions: mental arithmetic, stress film and cold pressor. Each session consisted of one stressful task and one or two non-stressful (neutral) tasks. Following seven respiratory parameters were calculated from pneumotachograph recording: (1) breath time, (2) inspiratory time, (3) expiratory time, (4) post expiration pause time, (5) inspiratory volume, (6) expiratory volume, and (7) minute ventilation. There have been a few studies conducting the analysis of post-expiration pause time [7, 8]. Cohen et. al. [7] estimated pause time using inspiratory and expiratory peak amplitudes. Because this method for estimating pause time was lacking in accuracy when expiratory flow rate changed during expiration, pause time was calculated by the amount of time when expiratory flow rate drop to 100 ml per second in our studies [5, 6]. The analysis of the data showed that respiratory parameters showing constant change to different stressors were minute ventilation and post expiration pause time. As shown in Fig. 2, minute ventilation significantly increased and pause time significantly decreased to three different stressors. The data suggested that respiratory activity under stress is characterized by facilitation of ventilation and tends to be hyperventilated. Minute ventilation and pause time also showed significant changes to neutral stimulus. These two respiratory parameters mark a relaxation response since they responded to mild psychological stimuli.

Effect of stress on central respiratory mechanisms

Minute ventilation, the product of tidal volume (Vt) and respiration rate (RR), can be separated into respiratory dive and timing components according to the equation: $MV=VT \times RR=IV/IT \times IT/BT$ (BT: breath time, IT: inspiratory time, IV: inspiratory volume, respectively). The parameter IV/IT, an inspiratory flow rate, is commonly regarded as an index of the intensity of the "driving mechanism" and IT/BT represents "timing mechanism" [9]. Clark and von Euler [10] studied on changes of timing and drive during rebreathing, in cat and in man. They clarified that accumulation of CO_2 during rebreathing produced increased inspiratory flow rate (drive) but did not affect on duty cycle (timing). Recently, we have conducted some experiments to reveal effects of psychological stress on respiratory central mechanisms [11, 12]. Time and drive components were determined on a breath-by-breath basis by using pneumotachograph recording. Twenty

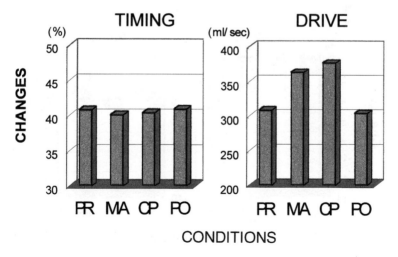

Fig. 3. Indices of respiratory timing (left) and drive (right) during pre-rest (PR), mental arithmetic (MA), the cold pressor test (CP), and post-rest (PO)

healthy male and female undergraduates participated in the experiment consisted of mental arithmetic (active coping task) and cold pressor (passive coping). As shown in Fig. 3, an index of respiratory drive showed significant increases during mental arithmetic and cold pressor, whereas an index of respiratory timing did not show any significant changes. This finding was replicated in another experiment [12], in which thirty male and female subjects experienced mental arithmetic and a video game. An index of drive increased during mental arithmetic and a video game, whereas an index of timing did not show any constant changes during both stressors. The results obtained in two experiments suggested that psychological stress influenced the respiratory drive mechanism dominantly and that the respiratory timing mechanism is maintained to be stable during stress. The results also suggested that respiratory changes under stress are similar with changes observed in rebreathing manipulation, and that respiratory center acts during stress as if elevation in $PaCO_2$ did occur.

Effect of stress on gas exchange system

It is well known that the respiratory center control the partial pressure of CO_2 in arterial blood ($PaCO_2$) within 2-3 mmHg during one day [13]. There are the two noninvasive $PaCO_2$ monitors used most commonly, one of which is fractional end-tidal CO_2 ($petCO_2$) monitoring, and the other of which is transcutaneous pCO_2 ($tcpCO_2$) monitoring. In respiratory psychophysiology, several studies measured $petCO_2$ to estimate $PaCO_2$ and reported that psychological stress produced decrement in $petCO_2$ [4, 14]. There have been, however, few studies in which $PaCO_2$ is estimated by $tcpCO_2$ which is considered to be a consistently accurate reflection of $PaCO_2$ [15]. Therefore we conducted one experiment to clarify the effects of stress on gas exchange by using $tcpCO_2$ monitoring. Twenty male and female subjects participated the following experimental sessions: mental arithmetic, cold pressor, hyperventilation, and breath-holding. Continuous monitoring of pneumotachograph, $petCO_2$, $tcpCO_2$, electrocardiogram and arterial blood pressure, were carried out with subjects in the supine position. Analyzing data replicated that minute ventilation, inspiratory flow rate (drive), mean blood pressure, and heart rate significantly increased under both stressors. As shown in the left side of Fig. 4, $petCO_2$ significantly decreased during mental arithmetic and cold pressor. The absolute decrements in $petCO_2$ under mental arithmetic and cold pressor were -1.52 mmHg and -3.08 mmHg, respectively. These decrements

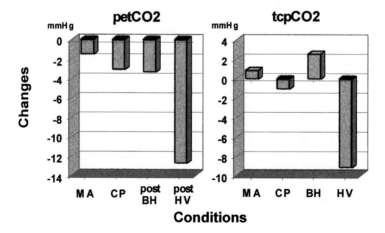

Fig. 4. Mean changes in end-tidal pCO_2 during MA, CP, postBH and postHV (left), whereas mean changes in transcutaneous pCO_2 during each condition (right).

were coincident with ones reported by other studies [4, 14]. As shown in the right side in Fig. 4, the changes in tcpCO2 during mental arithmetic and cold pressor were +1.2 mmHg and -1.1 mmHg, respectively. Significant decrement in tcpCO2 was observed in cold pressor condition only. The absolute decrement in tcpCO2 under cold pressor was significantly smaller than one in petCO2. To resolve the discrepancy between petCO2 and tcpCO2, changes in petCO2 and tcpCO2 during- and post- hyperventilation and breath-holding were analyzed. The mean changes in tcpCO2 under the hyperventilation and breath-holding conditions, were −9.17 mmHg and 2.53 mmHg, respectively. These data suggested that tcpCO2 correctly reflected changes in PaCO2. However mean changes in petCO2 after hyperventilation and breath-holding were −12.74 mmHg and −3.37 mmHg, respectively. Further analysis revealed that changes in respiration rate was negatively correlated with changes in petCO2 (r=-.68, p=.0012) and positively correlated with changes in tcpCO2 (r=.31, ns), which suggested that decrement in petCO2 was lacking in accuracy when respiration rate increased. Several studies reported that decrement in petCO2 during stress, and conclude that hyperventilation is the typical stress-associated respiratory changes [14, 16]. However, results of our recent studies suggested that minute ventilation and respiratory drive are facilitated by stress but PaCO2 estimated by tcPCO2 is maintained to be stable during stress, and also suggested that respiratory system has sub-system sensitive to stress and another sub-system stable under stress.

Cardiorespiratory reactivity and individual characteristic of alexithymia

There is a large individual difference on respiratory reactivity to psychological stress. For example, respiration rate during mental arithmetic varied from 10 cycles per minute (cpm) to 30 cpm. Recently we studied on the relationship between cardiorespiratory reactivity and individual characteristic of alexithymia [17]. A principal characteristic of alexithymia is represented by the difficulty in expressing emotions verbally, a personality trait observed in classical psychosomatic patients [18]. Previous studies were unclear as to the relationship between physiological reactivity to stress and alexithymia. Although some studies indicated that high alexithymic subjects experienced high physiological arousal [19], other studies pointed out that high alexithymic subjects showed low arousal [20]. Therefore, Umezawa, et. al. [21] attempted to clarify the

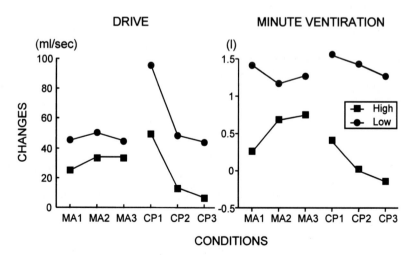

Fig. 5. Mean changes in drive (left) and minute ventilation (right) during mental arithmetic (MA) and cold pressor (CP) for high- and low- alexithymic groups

relationship between cardiorespiratory reactivity to laboratory stressors and alexithymia. Twenty-five healthy male and female undergraduate participants completed the 20-item Toronto Alexithymia Scale (TAS-20) [22] and the Minnesota Multiphasic Personality Inventory (MMPI). Participants were then divided into high- and low-alexithymic groups based on the median value of the TAS-20. Following a 20-min baseline rest, participants were asked to work on three mental arithmetic presentations, and on cold pressor test. Minute ventilation, mean flow rate (drive), heart rate and mean blood pressure increased significantly from baseline to mental arithmetic and cold pressor conditions, whereas an index of respiratory timing did not show any significant changes. High alexithymic group scored significantly higher on the MMPI F, D, Pa, Pt, and Sc scales. As shown in Fig. 5, however, increments in drive and minute ventilation from baseline for the high-alexithymic group significantly less than ones for the low-alexithymic group. Increments in respiration rate and heart rate for the high-alexithymic group under both stressors were also significantly less than ones for the low-alexithymic group. There was no significant difference in mean blood pressure between two groups. These results suggested that high-alexithymic subjects are more likely to have high subjective arousal and low cardiorespiratory reactivity against stressors, and also suggested that it should be difficult for high-alexithymic subjects to aware of emotion-associated bodily processes because physiological and somatic change being too small, which might cause difficulties to identify feelings.

Inhibitory breathing during detection of deception

Psychophysiological detection of deception is a method of determining when an individual is lying and it has a long history. In Japan most of polygraph examinations in field setting have been conducted by using the guilty knowledge test (GKT). The GKT involves some sub-tests, each consists of one critical question and several non-critical questions. A critical question contains specific information which identifiable only a criminal. If a suspect shows physiological reactivity to a critical question (CR) is greater then non-critical ones (nCR), he (or she) should have guilty knowledge [23]. It is well known that electrodermal response is more effective in discriminating deception than other physiological measures in laboratory setting. However Timm [24] maintained that respiration patterns are the most valid physiological indicators of deception in filed setting and that suppression of breathing to critical questions is indicative of deception. Timm proposed that an index of respiration line length (RLL) had detection efficiency, and that guilty suspects showed their greatest respiration suppression. RLL has been used in recent field and laboratory studies in which the shortest RLL is thought to be a marker of deception. Respiration is usually measured by bellows attached around subject's chest and abdomen. Therefore, it is difficult to quantitative analysis of ventilation without calibration procedure. There have been few studies showed that deception is accompanied with inhibition breathing by the quantitative measurement such as pneumotachograph. Deception accompanied with electrodermal response reflecting sympathetic nervous system. Since lie detection is a stressful situation for an individual, Therefore, it could be hypothesized that an index of respiratory drive should increase significantly even if tidal volume would decrease during deception.

To test this hypothesis, Kurohara et. al. [12] conducted the experiment to clarify the respiratory changes in the detection of deception and to compare the differences between respiratory changes under a mock-crime situation and under laboratory stress. Following 20 minutes adaptation period, 17 male and 13 female undergraduate students participated in the following three sessions: detection of deception, mental arithmetic and the video game. Subjects were instructed to conceal the critical item which they had previously selected in mock crime situation. The GKT was used as questioning technique in the detection of deception condition. Contrary to our expectations, we found that breathing patterns under the detection of deception situation was quite different from ones under stress. Fig. 6 shows that decrements in both expiratory volume and minute ventilation against critical questions (CR) were significantly greater than ones against non-critical ones. An index of respiratory drive did not show any significant changes. The result of this experiment

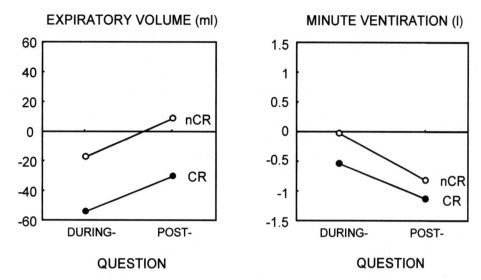

Fig. 6. Mean changes in expiratory volume (left) and minute ventilation (right) against critical (CR) and non-critical (nCR) questions.

clearly suggested that respiration during deception is characterized by inhibitory breathing nevertheless detection of deception is a stressful situation.

Ambulatory monitoring of respiration: Facilitation and inhibition of breathing in real life situation

As Boiten [8] pointed out, relationship between different emotions and respiration remains obscure because of some obstacles. A major obstacle is the difficulty in inducing real life emotion in a laboratory setting. Therefore, we attempted ambulatory monitoring of respiration to investigate the facilitation and inhibition of breathing in real life and to clarify links between emotion and breathing [25]. We conducted ambulatory monitoring of respiratory movements by using respiratory inductive plethysmography (RIP) and estimation of tidal volume (Vt) based on the sum of volume displacement of rib cage (RC) and abdomen (AB). Prior to the ambulatory measurement, subjects participated the 15 min. calibration procedure comparing with changes in respiratory movements measured by RIP to simultaneous pneumotachograph (PT) recording in the three body positions: supine, sitting and standing. The RC and the AB volume-motion coefficients were calculated from the data obtained in three body positions. The W_{RB} and W_{AB} values in the following formula were estimated by using the multiple regression analysis method. The intrasubject correlation coefficient between the estimated Vt (RIP) and the actual Vt (PT) standardizes 0.8 or more within the range of 500 ml. That prevents to get influenced by extremely a large and a small tidal volumes when a correlation was calculated. Correlation between the estimated Vt and the actual Vt values were more than .8 in all subjects.

$$Vt = W_{RB}\triangle RB + W_{AB}\triangle AB$$
$$W_{RB} + W_{AB} = 1$$

The weight of a RIP equipment and a digital data recorder used a PCMCIA flash memory card was totally 600 g. The equipment and the data recorder were put into a small bag attached to a subject's waist. Fig. 7 shows the overall changes in estimated minute ventilation by using RIP in the 6 hours ambulatory monitoring for one subject. A line in the graph illustrates a desk work. It was found that the estimated minute ventilation sometimes increased and sometime decreased compared with resting values pre- and post- of the ambulatory measurement even when a subject engaged a deskwork without gross body movements was done. Fig. 7 also suggests that respiration in real life situations was characterized by being compound of hyperventilation and hypoventilation. There have been different breath therapies one of which recommends slow and predominantly abdominal breathing and another of which recommended effortless breathing. Data of ambulatory breathing suggested that reducing irregularity of breathing will be one method for stress reduction in real life. In fact, von Dixhoorn [26] reported that breathing instruction, passive attention to spontaneous breathing and active regulation breathing, improved psychophysiological outcome of rehabilitation after myocardial infarction.

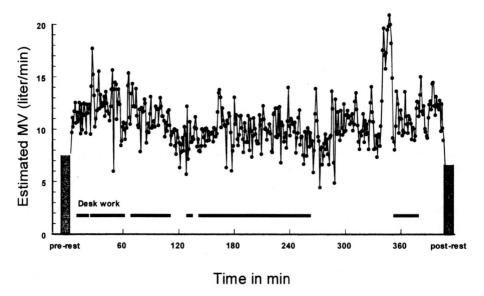

Fig. 7. The overall changes in estimated minute ventilation during the 6 hours ambulatory monitoring for one subject (male, 48 yrs.). Lines in the graph illustrates engaging himself in desk-working.

Conclusion

In summary, psychological stress influenced respiratory drive mechanism dominantly and respiratory timing and gas exchange were maintained stable during stress. In contradictory to our prediction, breathing during deception tended to be hypoventilated. Inhibitory breathing during deception is thought to be produced by influence from upper center to respiratory center, because the major difference between stress and detection of deception is whether conscious inhibition does occur or not. We also expect that conscious inhibition tend to occur in our emotional experience. Most of previous studies concerning about links between stress and respiration point out hyperventilation induced by stress but few studies reported on inhibitory breathing under stress. Exceptionally, Anderson [27] found that experimental animals exhibited mild, but sustained, inhibition of breathing preceding the onset of each avoidance performance session. As shown in Fig. 8, it could be hypothesized that emotion such as fear might take a significant part in producing inhibitory breathing during deception and pre-avoidance period reported by Anderson

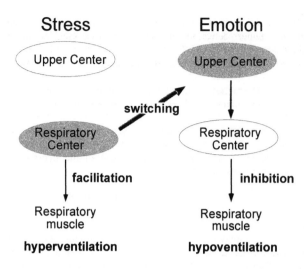

Fig. 8. The psychophysiological model on facilitation and inhibition of breathing during emotion and stress.

[27]. Additional studies are needed to clarify which psychological factors cause inhibitory breathing. These studies are expected to make great contribution to the psychophysiological study on emotion.

References

1. Umezawa A (1997) Self-regulation of respiratory activities in real life situations: Ambulatory monitoring of ventilation using respiratory movements. Japanese Biofeedback Research 24: 22-27
2. Ishikawa H, Kikuchi T (1977) A study on respiratory biofeedback. Japanese Journal of Behavior Therapy 3: 26-33
3. Benson H, Beary F, Carol MP (1974) Relaxation response. Psychiatry 37:37-46
4. Wientjes CJE, Grossman P, Gaillard AWK (1998) Influence of drive and timing mechanisms on breathing pattern and ventilation during mental task performance. Biological Psychology 49: 53-70
5. Umezawa A (1991) Changes of respiratory activity during laboratory stress. Japanese Journal of Physiological Psychology and Psychophysiology 9:43-55
6. Umezawa A (1992) Effects of stress on post-expiratory pause time and minute ventilation volume. In: Shirakura K, Saito I, Tutsui S (eds) Current biofeedback research in Japan. Shikoh Igaku Shuppan, Tokyo, pp125-132
7. Cohen HD, Goodenough DR, Witkin, HA Oltman P, Gould H, Shulman E (1975) The effects of stress on components of the respiration cycle. Psycho-physiology 12:377-380
8. Boiten FA (1998) The effects of emotional behaviour on components of the respiratory cycle. Biological Psychology 49: 29-51
9. Milic-Emili J, Grunstein MM (1976) Drive and timing components of ventilation. Chest 70: 131-133
10. Clark FJ, von Euler C (1972) On the regulation of depth and rate of breathing. Journal of Physiology 222: 267-295
11. Umezawa A (1999) Effect of stress on the central respiratory mechanisms and gas exchange. Psychophysiology 36(Suppl. 1):S61

12. Kurohara A, Terai K, Takeuchi H, Umezawa (1999) Changes in central respiratory timing and drive mechanisms under detection of deception. Japanese Journal of Physiological Psychology and Psychophysiology 17:75

13. West, J. B. (1995) Respiratory Physiology: the essentials. 5th ed. Williams & Wilkins, Baltimore

14. Ley R, Yelich G (1998) Fractional end-tidal CO_2 as an index of the effects of stress on math performance and verbal memory of test-anxious adolescents. Biological Psychology 49: 83-94

15. Pilsbury D, Hibbert GA (1987) An ambulatory system for long-term continuous monitoring of transcutaneous PCO_2. Bulletin of Europeen de Physiopathologie Respiratoire 23: 9-13

16. Garssen B (1980) Role of stress in the development of the hyperventilation syndrome. Psychotherapy and Psychosomatics 33:214-225.

17. Takeuchi H, Terai K, Umezawa A (1999) Effects of stress on the cardiovascular reactivity and individual characteristic alexithymia. Japanese Biofeedback Research 26: (in press)

18. Sifneos PE (1973) The prevalence of 'alexithymic' characteristic in psychosomatic patients. Psychotherapy and Psychosomatics 22: 255-262

19. Wehmer F, Brejnak C, Lumley M, Stettner L (1995) Alexithymia and physiological reactivity to emotion-provoking visual scenes. Journal of Nervous and Mental Disease 183: 351-357

20. Roedema MR, Simons FR (1999) Emotion-processing deficit in alexithymia. Psychophysiology 36: 379-387

21. Umezawa A, Terai K, Takeuchi H (1999) Cardiorespiratory reactivity under stress and individual caharacteristic of alexithymia. Biological Psychology (in press)

22. Bagby RM, Perker JDA, Taylor GJ (1994) The twenty-item toronto alexithymia scale-I. Item selection and cross-validation of the factor structure. Journal of Psychosomatic Research 38: 23-32

23. Lykken DT (1974) Psychology and the lie detector industry. American Psychologist 29: 725-739.

24. Timm HW (1982) Analyzing deception from respiration patterns. Journal of Police Science and Administration 10: 47-51

25. Umezawa A, Kuhorara A (1997) Ambulatory monitoring of respiratory activities in real daily life situations. Psychophysiology 34(Suppl. 1):S91

26. van Dixhoorn J (1999) Cariorespiratory effects of breathing and relaxation instruction in myocardial infarction patients. Biological Psychology 49:123-135

27. Anderson DE (1998) Cardiorenal effects of behavioral inhibition of breathing. Biological Psychology 49: 151-163

ENVIRONMENTAL STRESS, HYPOVENTILATORY BREATHING AND BLOOD PRESSURE REGULATION

David E. Anderson

Laboratory of Cardiovascular Science, National Institute on Aging, 5600 Nathan Shock Drive, Baltimore, MD 21224, USA

SUMMARY

Research in our laboratory is based on the hypothesis that chronic breathing suppression associated with stressful environments can contribute to high blood pressure via its effects on pCO_2, acid-base balance, and renal regulation of sodium. This hypothesis first emerged in the context of studies that investigated the role of behavioral stress in the development of experimental hypertension in laboratory animals. Those studies showed that regular exposure of animals to familar avoidance tasks evoked an anticipatory hypoventilatory breathing pattern associated with sustained increases in pCO_2. Repeated evocation of this breathing pattern potentiated the development of experimental hypertension when combined with high sodium intake. Subsequent studies of ambulatory monitoring of human breathing showed that people also engage in episodes of breathing inhibition in the natural environment. Experimental studies found that when hydrated humans voluntarily decreased breathing frequency and thereby increased pCO_2, they retained sodium and increased plasma volume. It was hypothesized that humans with high resting pCO_2 might show the same blood pressure sensitivity to high sodium intake as observed in the animal studies in which pCO_2 was increased via behavioral stress. This hypothesis was confirmed in two experimental studies, suggesting that high resting pCO_2 might be a useful clinical marker for sodium sensitivity. Recent studies have also found that older women with high resting end tidal CO_2 tend to have higher resting systolic blood pressure than other women with lower resting end tidal CO_2. Additional studies are needed to further clarify the role of breathing habits in pCO_2 regulation and its role in blood pressure adaptations to high sodium diet.

BACKGROUND

Epidemiological studies support the view that environmental and behavioral factors can play a role in the development of hypertension. The relative societal prevalence of hypertension has been positively correlated with high sodium intake, low potassium intake, and other dietary variables [1]. In addition, when individuals from less developed cultures migrated to urban environments, their vulnerability to hypertension increased [2]. It is probable that changes in dietary patterns interact with societal stresses, since cloistered nuns whose blood pressure was followed longitudinally for 20 years showed a very low incidence of hypertension, relative to a matched control group of women living in urban environments who were on comparable diets [3]. Studies showing that a deficiency in the expression of emotion [4], generally, or inhibition

149

of anger [5], specifically, are linked with high blood pressure also indicate that certain behavioral interaction styles might mediate the development of hypertension.

It is often assumed that environmental conditions impact on blood pressure via effects on the sympathetic nervous system, but it is also possible that stress-induced changes in breathing patterns participate in the pathogenesis of this most common cardiovascular disorder. The following review presents findings that support the view that chronic suppression of breathing could increase blood pressure sensitivity to high sodium intake via effects on circulating carbon dioxide, acid-base balance, and renal sodium regulation, that might be independent of renal sympathetic activity. First, studies of experimental hypertension in laboratory animals are reviewed, showing the origins of this hypothesis. Then, observational and experimental studies with human subjects are described, which show that breathing inhibition occurs in the natural environment and that inhibition of breathing produces a cascade of physiological effects that can influence body sodium balance. Finally, data are presented which indicate that humans whose set point for pCO_2 is high are both "salt sensitive" and tend to have higher resting blood pressure as they age.

STRESS-INDUCED HYPOVENTILATION IN LABORATORY ANIMALS

Numerous studies with laboratory animals have shown that a contingency on behavior that involves active interactions with the external environment to avoid aversive stimuli is associated with activation of the sympathetic nervous system, which increases heart rate and cardiac output, and increases blood pressure acutely.[e.g 6]. Under these conditions, animals increase ventilation to match the increased oxygen consumption. This "fight or flight" reaction has often been suggested as one way in which stress might participate in the development of chronic hypertension. It is less well known that when an animal is also confined in the experimental environment for a fixed period of time (an hour or more) preceding each daily avoidance performance session, an anticipatory cardiorespiratory response emerges, consisting of gradual and progressive decreases in respiration rate below resting levels, together with progressive increases in total peripheral resistance that maintain or increase blood pressure. This cardiorespiratory pattern emerges as the animal quietly awaited the stimulus signaling the onset of the avoidance session.

This anticipatory response is similar to the "orienting" reflex described by Pavlov, which occurs when an animal is exposed to an unexpected, novel stimulus [7]. With repeated exposure to the stimulus, that reflex diminishes, and then ceases to be elicited by the no longer novel stimulus. In animals in pre-avoidance periods, however, the situation has information value regarding the imminence of occurrence of behaviorally-relevant stimuli, and this "vigilance" response continues to be observed session after session, without diminution. The progressive respiratory suppression preceding the onset of avoidance sessions has been shown to be associated with sustained increases in pCO_2 [6,8]. pCO_2 was found to be higher during the pre-avoidance periods than at rest or during performance of the avoidance task. Plasma pH was lower during the early part of the pre-avoidance period than in the home kennel, but recovered to resting levels by the end of the pre-avoidance period. The changes in plasma pH reflected increases in hydrogen ion concentrations, due to increases in formation of, and dissociation of, carbonic acid from the combination of water and carbon dioxide. Plasma bicarbonate concentrations increased progressively during the pre-avoidance and avoidance periods, compared with resting controls, helping to restore normal pH.

Plasma concentrations of endogenous digitalis-like factors (EDLF) were analyzed to provide information on changes in plasma volume under these conditions. These factors have been shown to have both natriuretic and vasoconstrictor properties, due to inhibition of the sodium-potassium pump in the kidneys and vascular smooth muscle, respectively [9]. Plasma EDLF were increased at the end of pre-avoidance periods and during the avoidance sessions, compared with levels in the home kennel and at the beginning of the pre-avoidance sessions. These responses indicate that plasma volume expanded during the pre-avoidance periods, presumably because the slow infusion of saline to maintain catheter patency was not matched by proportional excretion of sodium by the kidneys. In these studies, erythrocyte sodium-potassium pump activity was suppressed during pre-avoidance periods, but was not suppressed during the avoidance sessions. Thus, the effects of EDLF on vascular tone and blood pressure depend on concurrent concentrations of other vasoconstrictor or vasodilator hormones also elicited by the environmental demands.

Ordinarily, the blood pressure of most animals is resistant to high sodium intake, since the kidneys maintain body sodium balance by excreting salt in proportion to the rate at which it is ingested. However, when animals were maintained on schedules that maintained the pre0-avoidance patterns, their 24-hour mean blood pressure increased over periods of days, if , and only if, isotonic saline was continuously infused into the circulation (at levels that were equivalent to the upper end of the human dietary range of salt intake) [10]. This form of hypertension did not develop in animals who received the saline infusion in the absence of behavioral stress, and did not develop under conditions of behavioral stress with normal sodium intake. It was associated with sustained renal sodium retention [10] and could be reversed by increases in 24-hr potassium intake [11]. However, it was not prevented by either renal denervation or adrenergic antagonists [12], suggesting that renal sympathetic nervous system activity was not responsible for the sodium retention and blood pressure elevation. Thus, an experimental procedure was developed that reliably produced hypertensive adaptations via a specific respiratory effect of behavioral stress that compromised the ability of the kidneys to autoregulate body sodium levels.

INHIBITED BREATHING IN HUMANS: OBSERVATIONAL AND EXPERIMENTAL STUDIES

Do humans show respiratory suppression in the natural environment similar to that in laboratory animals under conditions of behavioral stress? The oft heard injunction "don't hold your breath" regarding the probability of some future event suggests that we do. However, it is difficult to objectively study human breathing in the natural environment over extended time periods, because, although breathing is rhythmic at rest, it can be irregular in both frequency and depth during active behavior, and the quantitation of breathing frequency and depth becomes problematic. An attempt to solve this problem was made by development of an ambulatory monitor of breathing. The technology was based on the principle that expansion of elasticized bands around the chest and abdomen during inspiration is proportional to the inspirational volume [13]. Earlier studies had shown that inductive plethysmography provided a reasonably accurate measure of tidal volume in seated [14], exercising [15] and sleeping [16] individuals. The portable microprocessor recorded tidal volume of each breath, and counted breaths over successive 10-minute intervals [17]. The microprocessor contained filters to delete inductance changes caused by non-respiratory movements. One filter was based on the observation that humans breathe about once every four seconds, but almost never as fast as once every two seconds (i.e. 30 breaths per minute). Thus, all chest movements occurring within two sec of a previous breath were excluded, thereby eliminating approximately 50% of all possible artifact. A second filter was based on the observation that chest expansion associated with breathing shows a maximum that is far below that which can be observed with some postural changes. Thus, any chest expansion above a certain level was also automatically screened out. This would leave only extraneous chest movements occurring in the range of the breathing depth and near the time that a breath would normally occur. Pilot observations showed that individual differences in 24-hr breathing patterns could be discerned readily with this technology.

Initial studies with the monitor showed that, as expected, mean tidal volume and minute ventilation were consistently higher during the daytime than at night [18]. However, mean breathing frequency was not greater during the day than at night, because periods of lower frequency breathing during the day offset periods of higher frequency breathing. Thus, the standard deviation of tidal volume was greater during the day than at night, corresponding to behavioral activation or inhibition, respectively. Periods of low frequency (or suppressed) breathing during the day occurred in a context of normal (not increased) tidal volume, indicating that those were also periods of low ventilation, and presumably, decreased oxygen consumption. Inhibited breathing was found to be more likely to occur when subjects were with others than when they were alone, and was more likely to occur at work than at home [19]. The breathing suppression appeared to be distinct, therefore, from respiratory concomitants of speaking, which, in any case, is typically associated with increases in minute ventilation [20]. Systolic blood pressure (but not heart rate) tended to be higher during episodes of inhibited breathing than at other times [21]. We concluded that the kind of breathing suppression that can be produced experimentally in laboratory animals also occurs "spontaneously" in humans in their natural environments.

The previously cited animal studies suggested that breathing inhibition might be important for blood pressure regulation due to effects on pCO_2 and acid-base balance. However, decreases in breathing frequency or depth will increase pCO_2 only if they are not accompanied by corresponding decreases in metabolic production of CO_2. We wanted to investigate whether suppression of breathing in humans which increased pCO_2 would have effects on renal sodium excretion that were similar to those observed in the animal studies. A laboratory task was devised that required each subject to breathe into a respiratory gas monitor that provided digital, breath-to-breath feedback of end tidal CO_2, which tends to be a few mmHg lower than pCO_2, but to covary with it. Each subject was instructed to increase end tidal CO_2 as high as could be comfortably sustained by decreasing breathing frequency at a normal tidal volume. Performance of this task required concentration and practice, but virtually all subjects learned to increase end tidal CO_2 by several mmHg above resting levels, which for most subjects range from 36 to 39 mmHg.

In one study [22], the experimental procedure consisted of a 10 min baseline period of normal breathing with no feedback, followed by a 15 min period of task breathing with feedback, followed by a 10 min recovery period with no feedback. Blood samples were collected every 5 min during these experiments via a venous catheter. Performance of the breathing task was found to be associated with sustained increases in pCO_2, decreases in plasma pH, and gradual increases in plasma bicarbonate concentrations, compared with a preceding baseline interval of normal breathing, and these effects were reversed during a 10 min recovery period. The same patterns were elicited whether end tidal CO_2 was elevated by low frequency/normal tidal volume or by low tidal volume/normal frequency breathing. Leg muscle sympathetic nerve activity recorded via micro-neurography was found to remain stable during task breathing [23]. In another study [24], subjects ingested water according to an established protocol [25] to increase rates of urine flow during performance of the breathing task. Urine samples were collected after 30 min normal breathing (baseline), after 30 min of task (hypoventilatory) breathing, and after 30 min of normal breathing (recovery). Urine volume and sodium excretion were decreased during hypoventilatory breathing, compared with the normal breathing periods of baseline and recovery, while urinary concentrations of EDLF were increased within 30 min after the breathing task. This study indicates that hypoventilatory breathing can retard renal excretion of sodium and water, and can expand plasma volume. Another study [26] investigated the effects of task breathing on plasma EDLF and erythrocyte sodium/potassium pump activity. EDLF are known to compete with potassium for the receptor site on the sodium-potassium ATPase on cell membranes, and if EDLF are increased, sodium/potassium pump activity should be decreased. Inhibition of sodium/potassium pump activity would tend to increase sodium excretion but also increase vascular tone. In this study, a venous catheter was implanted to obtain blood samples after a 15 min baseline period, a 30 min task period, and a 20 min recovery period. Plasma EDLF increased during task breathing and decreased to baseline levels during the recovery period. Consistent with this, erythrocyte sodium/potassium pump activity was inhibited during task breathing. Those subjects with the highest end tidal CO_2 were found to have the lowest erythrocyte sodium/potassium pump activity at rest [27], suggesting the possibility that high pCO_2 is a marker for high relative plasma volume. These findings provide further evidence that hypoventilatory breathing elicits changes in plasma volume and vascular tone, and raises the possibility that chronically high resting pCO_2 might be accompanied by chronically high levels of plasma volume.

INDIVIDUAL DIFFERENCES IN RESTING END TIDAL CO_2 AND SODIUM SENSITIVITY IN HUMANS

People show relatively large individual differences in resting end tidal CO_2, and these differences tend to be relatively stable over time [28]. In addition, individual resting end tidal CO_2 has been linked to a personality trait. When the NEO Personality Inventory was administered to a group of healthy humans, no associations of end tidal CO_2 with the Extraversion, Openness, Agreeableness or Conscientiousness scales were observed. However, there was a striking positive association of end tidal CO_2 with the Neuroticism Scale, which assesses the tendency to worry and experience negative emotions [28]. This findings of an association between the resting end tidal CO_2 and emotional state in humans, on the one hand, and acute increases in pCO_2 during behavioral stresses, on the other, led to the hypothesis that high resting end tidal CO_2 might be a consequence of habitual breathing suppression and might be associated with increased blood pressure sensitivity to high sodium intake in humans, as well as animals. It was already established that a decreased ability of the kidneys to excrete sodium characterizes humans with salt sensitivity [29], but the origins of this deficit are not known.

Previous research has shown that blood pressure sensitivity to high sodium intake is greater in older, than in younger, humans [30]. We conducted a study with normotensive men and women, ages 40-70, whose resting blood pressure was measured in the laboratory and whose ambulatory blood pressure was measured hourly in the natural environment for 24 hr via before and after seven days of high sodium intake [31]. Dietary intake of sodium was standardized by avoidance of high sodium foods ("fast" foods, frozen commercial dinners, processed meats, salted snack foods, canned soups and pasta, and table and cooking salt) and increased by ingestion of enteric-coated sodium chloride capsules. Two servings of fruits or vegetables were scheduled daily to standardize intake of potassium. Adherence to the diet was determined by monitoring overnight urinary sodium and potassium excretion. Urinary excretion of EDLF was also measured before and after high sodium intake in this study. The high sodium diet was associated with increased urinary sodium excretion and body weight. The high sodium diet produced significant increases in resting and 24-hr ambulatory systolic blood pressure in the highest two CO_2 quartiles only, and increases in diastolic blood pressure in the highest CO_2 quartile only. Subjects with high resting end tidal CO_2 showed higher levels of EDLF, both before and after sodium loading.

A second study was conducted with younger normotensive men and women, who tend to be much less salt sensitive [32]. No significant effects of sodium loading were observed on systolic or diastolic blood pressure for the younger group, as a whole. However, significant positive associations were found between individual mean resting $PetCO_2$ and the changes in individual resting systolic and diastolic blood pressure. The high $PetCO_2$ subjects showed no significant changes in systolic or diastolic blood pressure, but the lower $PetCO_2$ subjects showed significant decreases in systolic and diastolic blood pressure. The high $PetCO_2$ subjects showed a significant increase in ambulatory systolic blood pressure, while no change was observed in the lower group. Sodium loading increased mean urinary EDLF excretion in the younger group. A significant positive correlation was observed between individual mean $PetCO_2$ and the change in urinary EDLF excretion following sodium loading.

It has long been thought (though never proven) that people whose blood pressure is sensitive to high sodium intake are more likely to develop chronic hypertension as they age. pCO_2 of men is known to decrease with age [33], but no studies of age-associated changes in end tidal CO_2 of women are available. We conducted a cross-sectional study of age-associated changes in end tidal CO_2 of 313 healthy male and female participants in the Baltimore Longitudinal Study on Aging [34]. Exclusion criteria included a history of cardiovascular, pulmonary or related diseases and cigarette smoking. $PetCO_2$ was monitored continuously for 25 min from a nasal cannula attached to a respiratory gas monitor. Resting blood pressure was recorded every five minutes via an automated oscillometric device.

End tidal CO_2 of men decreased linearly over the life span. However, end tidal CO_2 of women remained stable across the life span. Mean end tidal CO_2 of young men was higher that of women, but mean end tidal CO_2 of women was higher than that of men. The findings for men replicate those for pCO_2 of men. The reasons for the gender difference in age-associated changes in end tidal CO_2 are not known, but are not due to differences in age-associated changes in pulmonary capacity, as measured by forced expiratory volume. Estrogen has been shown to decrease end tidal CO_2 [35], so the decreases in estrogen concentrations in women following menopause might counteract whatever factors operate to decrease end tidal CO_2 with age in men. Higher levels of estrogen have been associated with decreased blood pressure sensitivity to high dietary sodium intake [36]. It is of interest, therefore, that at least one study has found that sodium sensitivity of older women is greater than that of older men [37].

Finally, we investigated the role of end tidal CO_2 in resting blood pressure in men and women in the BLSA. Multiple regression analysis showed that end tidal CO_2 was a significant predictor of systolic blood pressure in women, which was independent of the effects of age or body mass index. This relationship was more striking after age 50. No such relationship was observed in men. The origins of these gender differences are not known, but studies of the relationships of emotional states to breathing patterns in men and women may be instructive.

THEORY AND CONCLUSIONS

The studies reviewed above are consistent with the view that while acute environmental events stimulate the sympathetic nervous system to increase blood pressure acutely, more chronic conditions can engender a psychophysiological state of increased "vigilance" that has a cascade of physiological effects, including hypoventilatory breathing, that can alter renal regulation of sodium and affect blood pressure over the long term. This cascade is depicted in Figure 1. Specifically, breathing suppression results in increased levels of pCO_2 (but within the normal range and not sufficient to trigger chemoreceptor reflexes). The increase in pCO_2 causes a transient decrease in plasma pH. This change in acid-base balance stimulates the kidneys to eliminate the excess acid, but at a cost of increased renal reabsorption of sodium and water. The sodium retention results in an expansion of plasma volume. The increase in plasma volume stimulates the secretion of EDLF which has both natriuretic and vasoconstrictor properties. Although pH recovers within an hour, a higher level of plasma volume is maintained as long as the pCO_2 remains increased. The high relative plasma volume renders blood pressure susceptible to the effects of a high sodium diet. It is hypothesized, therefore, that at least one subset of sodium sensitive individuals are characterized by high resting pCO_2. It is further hypothesized that resting pCO_2 level is a function of chronic breathing habits, and, in particular, the inhibition of breathing associated with chronic behavioral stress. The epidemiological studies showing increases in hypertension prevalence in individuals who migrate from less developed to more urban cultures [2] might be mediated by effects of the more stressful environments on breathing habits and pCO_2. In addition, the association of inhibition in expression of emotion with high blood pressure [4] might be mediated by breathing suppression and high pCO_2. Many of the individual associations are well established in the physiology literature. What remains to be done is to determine whether the system interdependencies operate in synchrony in the intact organism to produce the effects observed in experimental studies and in some kinds of human

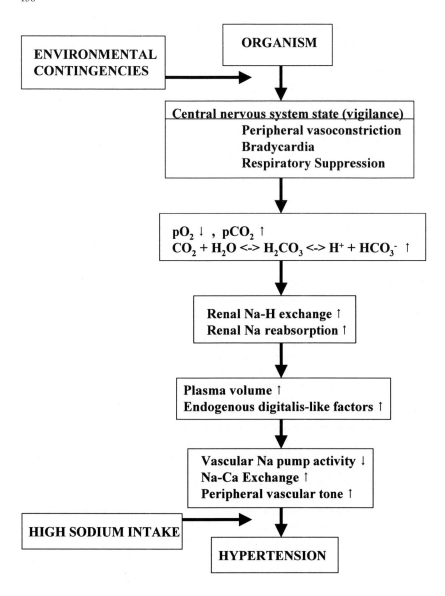

Figure 1. Cascade of physiological effects that occur within the context of hypoventilatory breathing during increased "vigilance" and their influence on blood pressure sensitivity to high sodium intake.

hypertension. From such studies may come understanding of the mechanisms by which adaptive breathing habits can have beneficial effects on blood pressure.

REFERENCES

1. Muntzel M, Drueke T. A comprehensive review of the salt and blood pressure relationships. American Journal of Hypertension, 1992, 5:S1-S42.

2. Poulter NR, Sever, PS. Low blood pressure populations and the impact of rural-urban migration. Swales JD (Ed) Textbook of Hypertension, Oxford:Balackwell, 1994, 22-35.

3.Timio M, Verdecchia P, Venanzi S, Gentli S, Roncoli M, Francucci B. Age and blood pressure changes. A 20 year followup study in nuns in a secluded order. Hypertension, 1988, 12, 457-461.

4. Jula A, Salminen JK, Saarijarvi S. Alexithymia: a facet of essential hypertension. Hypertension, 1999, 33:1057-1061.

5. Jorgensen RS, Johnson BT, Kolodziej ME, Schreer GE. Elevated blood pressure and personality: a meta-analytic review. Psychol. Bull, 1996; 120:293-320.

6. Anderson, D.E., Fedorova, O.V. & French, A.W. (1996) Hypercapnia and decreased hematocrit during preavoidance periods in the micropig. Physiology and Behavior, 1996 (in press)

7. Sokolov, EN. Perception and the conditioned reflex. Oxford:Pergamon Press, 1963.

8. Fedorova OV, French AW, Anderson DE. Inhibition of erythrocyte Na,K-ATPase activity during anticipatory hypoventilation in micropigs. *Am J Hypertens.* 1996;9:1126-1131

9. Bagrov, AY, Roukoyatkina N, Fedorova OV, Pinaev AG, Ukhanova MV. Digitalis-like and vasoconstrictor properties of endogenous digoxin-like factors from the venom of Bufo marinus toad. European Journal of Phramacology, 1993, 234:165-172.

10.Anderson DE. Experimental behavioral hypertension in laboratory animals. In Julius S, Bassett DR (Ed) Handbook of Hypertension. Vol 9. Amsterdam:Elsevier, 1987, pp 226-245.

11. Anderson DE, Kearns WD, Better WE. Potassium infusion attenuates avoidance-saline hypertension in dogs. Hypertension, 1983, 5, 415-419.

12. Anderson DE. Operant conditioning, sodium loading and experimental hypertension. Cardiovascular Pharmacol 1986; 8 (Suppl 5),:23-S30.

13. Konno K & Mead J. Measurement of the separate volume changes of rib cage and abdomen during breathing. Journal of Applied Physiology, 1967, 22, 407-422.

14. Cohn MA, Rao AS, Broudy M, Birch S, Watson H, Atkins N, Davis B, Scott FD & Sackner, MA. (1982) The respiratory inductive plethysmograph: a new non-invasive monitor of respiration. Bulletin of European Physiopathological Response, 18, 643-658.

15. Sackner JD Nixon AJ, Davis B, Atkins N, Sackner MA. (1980) Non-invasive measurement of ventilation during exercise using a respiratory inductive plethysmograph. American Journal of Respiratory Disease, 122:867-871.

16. Mason WJ, Kripke DF, Messin S & Ancoli-Isreal S (1986) The application and utilization of an ambulatory monitoring system for the screening of sleep disorders. American Journal of EEG Technology, 26:145-156.

17. Anderson, D.E. & Frank, L.B. (1990) A microprocessor-based system for monitoring breathing patterns in ambulatory subjects. Journal of Ambulatory Monitoring, 3, 11-20.

18. Anderson, D.E., Coyle, K. & Haythornthwaite, J.A. (1992) Ambulatory monitoring of respiration: inhibitory breathing in the natural environment. Psychophysiology, 29, 551-557.

19. Haythornthwaite, J.A., Anderson, D.E. & Moore, L.H. (1992) Social   and behavioral factors associated with episodes of inhibitory breathing. Journal of Behavioral Medicine, 15, 573-588.

20. Bunn, J.C. & Mead, J. (1971) Control of ventilation during speech. Journal of Applied Physiology, 31, 870-872.

21. Anderson, D.E., Austin, J.L. & Haythornthwaite, J.A. (1993) Blood pressure during sustained inhibitory breathing in the natural environment. Psychophysiology, 30, 131-137.

22. Anderson, D.E., Austin, J. & Coyle, K. (1993) Metabolic and hemodynamic effects of inhibitory breathing. Homeostasis, 34, 328-337.

23. Anderson, D.E., Somers, V.K., Clary, M.P. & Anderson, E. (1991) Sympathetic muscle nerve activity and hemodynamic responses during hypoventilation-induced hypercapnia in humans. Neuroscience Abstracts, 17, 201.

24. Anderson DE, Bagrov AY, Austin JL. Inhibited breathing decreases renal sodium excretion. *Psychosomatic Med.* 1995;57:373-380.

25. Light, K.C., Koepke, J.P., Obrist, P.A. & Willis, P.W. (1983) Psychological stress induced sodium and fluid retention in men at high risk for hypertension. Science 220:429-431.

26. Bagrov AY, Fedorova OV, Dmitrieva RI, Austin JL, Anderson DE. Endogenous marinobufagenin-like immunoreactive factor and Na,K-ATPase inhibition during voluntary hypoventilation. *Hypertension.* 1995;26:781-788.

27. Fedorova, O.V., Bagrov, A.Y., Austin-Lane, J.L. & Anderson, D.E. Na,K-ATPase inhibition during pressor response to hypoventilation. In Haunso, S. & Kjeldsen, K. (Eds)   International Society for Heart Research European Section Meeting XV. Bologna, Monduzzi editore, pp. 385-388.

28. Dhokalia, A, Parsons DJ, Anderson, DE. Resting end tidal CO_2 association with age, gender, and personality. Psychosom Med, 1998;60-33-37.

29. Zemel MB Sowers JR. Salt sensitivity and systemic hypertension in the elderly. American Journal of Cardiology, 1988, 61, 7H-12H.

30. Simamoto H, Shimamoto Y. Time course of hemodynamic responses to sodium in elderly hypertensive responses. Hypertension, 1990, 16, 387-397.

31. Anderson DE, Dhokalia A, Parsons DJ, Bagrov AY. High end tidal CO_2 association with blood pressure response to sodium loading in older adults. Journal of Hypertension, 1996, 14, 1073-1079.

32.Anderson DE, Dhokalia A, Parsons D, Bagrov AY Sodium sensitivity in yound adults with high resting end tidal CO_2 Journal of Hypertension, 1998, 16, 1015-1022.

33. Frassetto L, Sebastian A. Age and systemic acid-base equilibrium: analysis of published data. *J Gerontol.* 1996;51:691-699.

34. Anderson DE, Parsons DJ, Scuteri A. End tidal CO_2 is an independent determinant of systolic blood pressure in women. Journal of Hypertension, 1999, 17, 107301080.

35. Regensteiner JG, Woodward WD, Hagerman DD, Weil JV, Pickett CK, Bender PR. Combined effects of female hormones and metabolic rate on ventilatory drives in women. Journal of Applied Physiology 1989, 66, 808-813.

36. Tominaga T, Suzuki H, Ogata Y, Matsukawa S, Saruta T. The role of sex hormones and sodium intake in postmenopausal hypertension. Journal of Human Hypertension, 1991, 5, 495-500.

37. Nestel PJ, Clifton PM, Noakes M, MacArthur R, Howe PR. Enhanced blood pressure response to dietary salt in elderly women, especially those with small waist:hip ratio. Journal of Hypertension, 1993, 11:1387-1394.

Stress Reduction Intervention: A Theoretical Reconsideration with an Emphasis on Breathing Training

Yukihiro Sawada

Department of Psychology, School of Medicine, Sapporo Medical University, South 1 West 17, Chuo-ku, Sapporo, Hokkaido 060-8556, Japan (e-mail: sawaday@sapmed.ac.jp)

Summary: In recent years, considerable attention has been focused on studies of stress reduction interventions. However, there have been controversies regarding their positive effects. The present paper is an attempt to initiate reconciliation of the discrepant findings. First, the term "stress" is redefined from a standpoint of cardiovascular hemodynamics. Then the attention-affect model is newly introduced in order to have a clearer understanding of the hemodynamic reaction patterns during stressful stimulation. Based on these reconsiderations, the stress reduction interventions are revaluated, with an emphasis on breathing training.

Key words: Stress Reduction Intervention, Blood Pressure, Cardiovascular Hemodynamics, Attention, Unpleasant Affect

Some researchers have insisted that diaphragmatic breathing training can have therapeutic effects by influencing the cardiorespiratory system and daily moods such as anxiety [1]. However, there have been controversies regarding its positive effects [2, 3]. As will be discussed later, breathing training seems to be a mix of two kinds of stress reduction interventions: relaxation and meditation techniques; Accordingly, it is of importance to know how such stress reduction interventions as these, as well as biofeedback and cognitive approaches, can be therapeutically effective [4].

STRESS REDEFINED

Blood pressure (BP) as the desired value. As Julius (1988) has pointed out [5], the central nervous system, via the autonomic nervous system, mainly regulates blood pressure (BP), but not blood flow or resistance, in the cardiovascular system. That is, a certain level of BP is "desired" when confronting an environmental stimulus. This hypothesis could be validated from the evidence that BP does not change obviously before or after intravenous injection of alpha- or beta-blockers during exposure to a stressful stimulus, or during resting [6-9]. Alpha-blocker produces a drastic decrease in total vascular resistance but a simultaneous, compensatory increase in cardiac output. With the beta-blocker, just the reverse occurs: namely, a profound decrease in cardiac output compensated by augmented total vascular resistance. Eventually, in any case, BP will change, if at all, only to a small degree and be preserved at near the same level before and after the pharmacological manipulations.

Psychosocial pressor stimulus. According to this hypothesis, cardiovascular reactions to a variety of environmental stimuli should, first of all, be assessed through the degree of BP elevations (i.e., BP reactivity). Hereafter, a stimulus which evokes BP elevations will be referred to as a pressor stimulus. It can either be psychosocial or physical in its nature. However the latter is not our present concern because physical training, despite producing a temporal elevation in BP at the moment of training, has therapeutic effects by lowering BP after a long period of training. Thus a recurrent activation by a physical pressor stimulus does not seem to result in stress-related disease (e.g., hypertension).

Therefore, a psychosocial pressor stimulus, which has acute duration and mild-to-moderate strength, is well worth investigating. Almost all such stimuli can be seen as stressful. However, as can be recognized from Fig. 1, some of them cannot be considered as stressful in the common sense meaning of the word; for example, BP elevations when delighted with the win of a favorite baseball team. In this connection, it should also be noted that not a small part of the stressful stimuli would not raise BP. Nonetheless, a psychosocial pressor stimulus can be one of the most typical stressful stimuli which we undergo in the laboratory during a task and encounter in everyday life as an episode. In addition, it is important to bear in mind that a psychosocial pressor stimulus can be defined clearly from the BP reactions but a stressful stimulus has a wide range of usage as a term and cannot be defined uniformly (thus, shown as a dotted circle in Fig. 1).

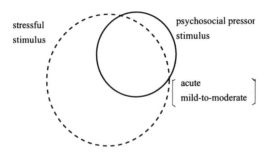

Fig. 1. Relation of psychosocial pressor stimulus on so-called stressful stimulus. The latter cannot be defined uniformly and thus is shwon as a dotted circle.

THE ATTENTION-AFFECT MODEL

Hemodynamic reaction pattern-I vs. -II. BP is a product of blood flow and resistance: mean BP= cardiac output X total peripheral resistance= (stroke volume X heart rate) X total peripheral resistance. Therefore, BP elevations to a psychosocial pressor stimulus result from increases in cardiac output and/or total peripheral resistance.

As shown in Table 1, BP elevations due to increases in cardiac output are typically accompanied by increases in heart rate and blood flow in the skeletal muscle and by both alpha- and beta-adrenergic sympathetic activations, as well as by vagal inhibition. In contrast, BP elevations due to increases in total peripheral resistance are accompanied by decreases in heart rate and blood flow in the skeletal muscle and by alpha- adrenergic sympathetic activation, as well as by slight vagal activation. These two types are referred to as hemodynamic reaction pattern-I and -II, respectively [10-12].

Active vs. passive coping. Recent studies have found that an important qualitative feature of the stimulus is whether it requires subjects to cope actively or passively [13]. In the active coping situation, subjects are usually asked to be challenging and/or competitive. On the other hand, subjects have little opportunity to escape stimulation and only tolerate in the passive coping situation. The findings have indicated that active coping would evoke elevations in BP via increases in cardiac output (i.e., pattern-I). In contrast, passive coping would produce elevations in BP through increases in total peripheral resistance (i.e., pattern-II) [6-9, 14-16].

Table 1. Two large groups of cardiovascular hemodynamics (pattern-I vs. II), as well as of their underlying autonomic activities a variety of stressful stimulation

	pattern-I	pattern-II
cardiovascular hemodynamics		
blood pressure	+	+
	(esp. systolic)	(esp. diastolic)
heart rate	+	−
cardiac output	+	−
muscle blood flow	+	−
activities	−	+
autonomic activities		
alpha-adrenergic sympathetic	+ *	+
bata-adrenergic sympathetic	+	−
vagal	−	+

* But, " − " in the muscle bood vessels

The attention-affect model. However, a body of evidence stands against the correspondence of pattern-I vs. -II to active vs. passive coping, respectively. One of the most clear pieces of counterevidence has been obtained from mirror drawing on a computer display. It superficially seems to require active coping but actually produces hemodynamic reaction pattern-II [17-19]. On the other hand, unavoidable exposure to shock, despite its passive coping nature, has resulted in pattern-I [20, 21].

The attention-affect model is newly developed in order to overcome these inconsistencies. As shown in Fig. 2, in this model it is postulated that cognitive appraisal of a psychosocial pressor stimulus primarily results in an unpleasant affect or in attention to the stimulus and subsequently that the hemodynamic reaction pattern-I or -II is produced according to the respective cognitive process. In addition, it is assumed that often an attention to performance or sometimes a pleasant affect could secondarily contribute to the respective pattern formation.

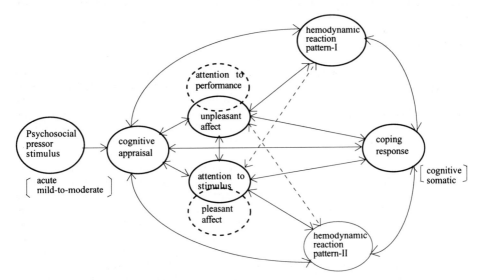

Fig. 2. The attention-affect model

The evidence of BP elevations via compensatory hemodynamic activations under alpha- or beta-blockers, as described above, is depicted by dotted arrows in Fig. 2. Coping response to a psychosocial pressor stimulus is more overwhelmingly cognitive than somatic in our modernized society (e.g., mental workload) and does not necessarily correspond to its hemodynamic reaction pattern.

The new model can explain without contradiction how both the stimulus which requires active coping (e.g., mental arithmetic; unpleasant affect plus attention to performance) and that which forces passive toleration (e.g., unavoidable exposure to shock; only an unpleasant affect) could converge to the same hemodynamic reaction pattern-I. In contrast, both the stimulus from which subjects have little opportunity to escape (e.g., noise; attention to stimulus and a bit of unpleasant affect) and that which requires active coping superficially (e.g., mirror drawing; attention to stimulus plus a bit of pleasant affect and a bit of unpleasant affect plus attention to performance) could result in the hemodynamic reaction pattern-II.

STRESS REDUCTION INTERVENTION

Plausible therapeutic mechanisms. Jacob and Chesney (1986) have listed relaxation and meditation techniques, as well as biofeedback and cognitive approaches, as possible candidates for stress reduction intervention [4]. And cardiovascular reactivities were checked for a variety of hemodynamic parameters (especially the heart rate). In the present context, however, stress reduction intervention can be defined as a group of nonpharmacologic techniques which can reduce BP elevations preceding, during, and/or following exposure to psychosocial pressor stimulus.

Given that the attention-affect model is valid, a reduction of BP elevations could be achieved primarily through a diminution of unpleasant affect or of attention to stimulus under hemodynamic reaction pattern-I or -II, respectively. Secondarily, a diminution of attention to performance or of pleasant affect could also be effective. Moreover, a modification of cognitive appraisal of the psychosocial pressor stimulus per se and/or a diminution of the hemodynamic reaction patterns themselves (especially, pattern-I) may be effective from a standpoint of the peripheral theory of emotion.

Specifically, breathing training can be seen as a mix of relaxation and meditation techniques prompting muscle and psychic tension relief and concentration on breathing rhythms. It may work by facilitating muscle and psychic relaxation, thereby counteracting the hightened muscle tension and unpleasant affect in hemodynamic reaction pattern-I. In addition, it may be efficacious because it occupies the subject's attention with breathing rhythms, making them less concerned with the unpleasant affect or with psychosocial pressor stimulus in the hemodynamic reaction pattern-I or -II, respectively. Moreover, the hemodynamic reaction patterns themselves may be affected by an alteration of acid-base balance through breathing training [22-24].

Previous findings. Given the perspective of the present report, only ten previous studies conducted with the aim of assessing stress reduction intervention are suitable for consideration [chronologically, 25-34]. In Fig. 3, only the %-change data on mean BP from resting baseline to an exposure to stressful stimulus are arranged in chronological order from the top left to bottom right, together with the authors' names and their reference numbers. Those before starting and after finishing the training of stress reduction intervention are shown as open and shaded bars, respectively, for both the training (T) and control (C) groups. A variety of stress reduction interventions are utilized in those ten studies: progressive relaxation (PR), biofeedback (BF), autogenic training (AT), yoga (YG), and breathing training (BrT, depicted in gothic letters). Cognitive approaches are scarcely utilized as a main intervention. With regard to a stressful task,

165

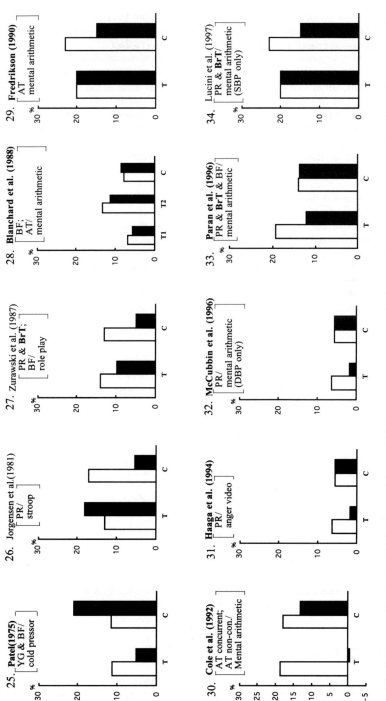

Fig. 3. Ten previous studies which presented data on blood pressure (BP) during stressful stimulation before strating and after finishing the training of stress reduction intervention (open and shaded bars, respectively). Here only percent change data on mean BP from resting baseline to an exposure to stressful stimulus are arranged in chronological order. The results by authors depicted in gothic letters are considered to be successful. T vs. C = training vs. control group. PR = progressive relaxation; BF = biofeedback; AT = authgenic traing; YG = yoga; BrT (in gothic) = breathing training.

mental arithmetic was utilized in most of the cases. The results by authors depicted in gothic letters are considered to be successful because a much shorter column length on the shaded bar than on the open one was found for T group as compared with C group.

Stress reducing effects were found in only some of the studies: diminished elevations in both the systolic and diastolic BP in four studies [25, 29-31], as well as those in the diastolic BP in three studies [28, 32, 33], during the exposure to psychosocial pressor stimulus. A reduction of BP elevations preceding or following the stimulus has seldom been demonstrated: only in two studies [26, 27] and one [25], respectively. Among the ten intervention studies, only three include breathing training (BrT) in their amalgam of techniques [27, 33, 34]. The results obtained were moderately effective as just mentioned above. In sum, however, it is difficult to draw any definitive conclusions.

It should be emphasized that relaxation and meditation techniques, as well as biofeedback and cognitive approaches, do not inevitably work as stress reduction interventions. For example, meditation will require the practitioner to dwell upon something in order to reduce mental distractions. However, it may fail to accomplish tension relief because of its high concentration on or mindfulness to the psychosocial pressor stimulus and/or to the unpleasant affect [35]. Accordingly, as can be seen in Fig. 4, these techniques should be viewed only as potential "candidates" for stress reduction intervention. Their positive effect has yet to be scientifically validated. With this in mind, it is hardly surprising that the previous studies just cited above achieved only moderate success in their attempts to verify their techniques.

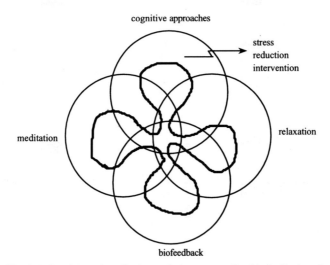

Fig. 4. Relaxation and meditation techniques, as well as biofeedback and cognitive approaches, as potential candidates for stress reduction intervention.

FUTURE DIRECTIONS

Assuming that the attention-affect model is adaptable to any kind of psychosocial pressor stimuli, it seems that it would be more appropriate to prescribe a specific stress reduction intervention against a specific psychosocial pressor stimulus. Breathing training is rather easy to practice for everyone and could be remarkably helpful to diminish an augmented hemodynamic reaction pattern-I or -II during any kind of stressful stimuli because of its mixed nature of relaxation and meditation techniques.

However, the previous studies, including those utilizing breathing training, have not tried to investigate systematically the hemodynamic reaction patterns of any techniques during, as well as preceding or following, exposure to stressful stimuli. Therefore, a reassessment of a variety of candidates for stress reduction interventions within the framework derived from the attention-affect model would seem to be worthwhile. Such an endeavor will enable us to confirm to what degree and through which mechanisms the traditional techniques or a newly developed one could exert their effects as a stress reduction intervention.

REFERENCES

1. Garssen B, de Ruiter C, van Dyck R (1992) Breathing retraining: A rational placebo? Clinical Psychology Review 12:141-153
2. Cappo BM, Holmes DS (1984) The utility of prolonged respiratory exhalation for reduced physiological and psychological arousal in non-threatening and threatening situations. Journal of Psychosomatic Research 28:265-273
3. Harris VA, Katkin ES, Lick JR, Habberfield T (1976) Paced respiration as a technique for the modification of autonomic response to stress. Psychophysiology 13:386-391
4. Jacob RG, Chesney MA (1986) Psychological and behavioral methods to reduce cardiovascular reactivity. In: Matthews KA, Weiss SM, Detre T, Dembroski TM, Falkner B, Manuck SB, Williams RB (eds) Handbook of stress, reactivity, and cardiovascular disease. John Wiley & Sons, New York, pp417-457
5. Julius S (1988) The blood pressure seeking properties of the central nervous system. Journal of Hypertension 6:177-185
6. Andrèn L (1982) Cardiovascular effects of noise. Acta Medica Scandinavica Suppl.657:1-45
7. Bonelli J, Hörtnagl H, Brücke Th, Magometschnigg D, Lochs H, Kaik G (1979) Effects of calculation stress on hemodynamics and plasma catecholamines before and after β - blockade with propranolol (Inderal ®) and mepindolol sulfate (Corindolan ®). European Journal of Clinical Pharmacology 15:1-8
8. Freyschuss U, Hjemdahl P, Juhlin-Dannfelt A, Linde B (1988) Cardiovascular and sympathoadrenal responses to mental stress: influence of β -blockade. American Journal of Physiology 255:H1443-H1451
9. Sherwood A, Allen MT, Obrist PA, Langer AW (1986) Evaluation of beta-adrenergic influences on cardiovascular and metabolic adjustments to physical and psychological stress. Psychophysiology 23:89-104
10. Williams RB (1986) Patterns of reactivity and stress. In: Matthews KA, Weiss SM, Detre T, Dembroski TM, Falkner B, Manuck SB, Williams RB (eds) Handbook of stress, reactivity, and cardiovascular disease. John Wiley & Sons, New York, pp109-125
11. Sawada Y (1990) Blood pressure reactivity: Construction of a series of hypotheses and their assessment. Japanese Psychological Review 33:209-238 (in Japanese with English summary)
12. Schneiderman N, McCabe PM (1989) Psychophysiologic strategies in laboratory research. In: Schneiderman N, Weiss SM, Kaufman PG (eds) Handbook of research methods in cardiovascular behavioral medicine. Plenum Press, New York, pp349-364
13. Obrist PA, Gaebelein CJ, Teller ES, Langer AW, Gringnolo A, Light KC, McCubbin JA (1978) The relationship between heart rate, carotid dP/dt, and blood pressure in humans as a function of the type of stress. Psychophysiology 15:102-115
14. Allen MT, Crowell MD (1989) Patterns of autonomic response during laboratory stressors. Psychophysiology 26:603-615
15. McKinney ME, Miner MH, Ruddel H, McIlvain HE, Witte H, Buell JC, Eliot RS, Grant LB

(1985) The standardized mental stress test protocol: Test-retest reliability and comparison with ambulatory blood pressure monitoring. Psychophysiology 22:453-463

16. Lovallo WR, Pincomb GA, Wilson MF (1986) Predicting response to a reaction time task: Heart rate reactivity compared with Type A behavior. Psychophysiology 23:648-656

17. Allen MT, Stoney CM, Owens JF, Matthews KA (1993) Hemodynamic adjustments to laboratory stress: The influence of gender and personality. Psychosomatic Medicine 55: 505-517

18. Hurwitz BE, Nelesen RA, Saab PG, Nagel JH, Spitzer SB, Gellman MD, McCabe PM, Phillips DJ, Schneiderman N (1993) Differential patterns of dynamic cardiovascular regulation as a function of task. Biological Psychology 36:75-95

19. Waldstein SR, Bachen EA, Manuck SB (1997) Active coping and cardiovascular reactivity: A multiplicity of influences. Psychosomatic Medicine 59:620-625

20. Lovallo WR, Pincomb GA, Wilson MF (1986) Heart rate reactivity and Type A behavior as modifiers of physiological response to active and passive coping. Psychophysiology 23:105-112.

21. Lovallo WR, Wilson MF, Pincomb GA, Edwards GL, Tompkins P, Brackett DJ (1985) Activation patterns to aversive stimulation in man: passive exposure versus effort to control. Psychophysiology 22:283-291

22. Anderson DE, Austin J, Coyle K (1993) Metabolic and hemodynamic effects of inhibitory breathing. Homeostasis 34:328-337

23. Grossman P (1983) Respiration, stress, and cardiovascular function. Psychophysiology 20:284-299

24. Sawada Y A preliminary study on a comfortable paced respiration. Japanese Psychological Research (in press)

25. Patel CH (1975) Yoga and biofeedback in the management of 'stress' in hypertensive patients. Clinical Science and Molecular Medicine 48:171s-174s

26. Jorgensen RS, Houston BK, Zurawski RM (1981) Anxiety management training in the treatment of essential hypertension. Behavior Research and Therapy 19:467-474

27. Zurawski RM, Smith TW, Houston BK (1987) Stress management for essential hypertension: Comparison with a minimally effective treatment, predictors of response to treatment, and effects on reactivity. Journal of Psychosomatic Research 31:453-462

28. Blanchard EB, McCoy GC, McCaffrey RJ, Wittrock DA, Musso A, Berger M, Aivasyan TA, Khramelashvili VV, Salenko BB (1988) The effects of thermal biofeedback and autogenic training of cardiovascular reactivity: The joint USSR-USA behavioral hypertension treatment project. Biofeedback and Self-Regulation 13:25-37

29. Fredrikson M (1990) Effects of autogenic training on cardiovascular and electrodermal reactivity to mental stress: an exploratory study. Journal of Psychophysiology 4:289-294

30. Cole PA, Pomerleau CS, Harris JK (1992) The effects of nonconcurrent and concurrent relaxation training on cardiovascular reactivity to a psychological stressor. Journal of Behavioral Medicine 15:407-4

31. Haaga DAF, Davison GC, Williams ME, Dolezal SL, Haleblian J, Rosenbaum J, Dwyer JH, Baker S, Nezami E, DeQuattro V (1994) Mode-specific impact of relaxation training for hypertensive men with Type A behavior pattern. Behavior Therapy 25:209-223

32. McCubbin JA, Wilson JF, Bruehl S, Ibarra P, Carlson CR, Norton JA, Colclough GW (1996) Relaxation training and opioid inhibition of blood pressure response to stress. Journal of Consulting and Clinical Psychology 64:593-601

33. Paran E, Amir M, Yaniv N (1996) Evaluating the response of mild hypertensives to biofeedback-assisted relaxation using a mental stress test. Journal of Behavior Therapy and Experimental Psychiatry 27:157-167

34. Lucini D, Covacci G, Milani R, Mela GS, Malliani A, Pagani M (1997). A controlled study of the effects of mental relaxation on autonomic excitatory responses in healthy subjects. Psychosomatic Medicine 59:541-552

35. Sawada Y, Steptoe A (1988) The effects of brief meditation training on cardiovascular stress responses. Journal of Psychophysiology 2:249-257

Special Lecture

Noh Theatre, The Aesthetics of Breathing

Naohiko Umewaka

Noh Master and Doctor of Philosophy in Drama, Royal Holloway University of London.
Shizuoka University of Art and Culture, Hamamatu, Shizuoka,   430-0919, Japan

It had always been in the breathing rhythm; this is where a weapon had been concealed. This concealed weapon could work dreadful impact.   The Samurai always possessed these two entirely different implements of destruction.   The visible and concealed weapon; these were the sword and breathing rhythm. Breathing rhythm as the implement of expression in Noh. This focus on breathing rhythm is not limited to Bushido, but holds true also for many of Japanese traditional performing arts.   Experts and the greatest thespians of Noh, one of Japanese most acclaimed performing arts, in particular had focused on breathing rhythm as an implement of expression for the past several hundred years.   They discovered that the body expression could be altered by breathing method and succeeded in incorporating breathing rhythm as an artistic element of their craft.   We Noh actors believe that in order to alter the outward expression of the body, we ourselves must consciously stir change in composure of the body internal, feel the sensation of transformation while at the same time let the body itself speak as a means of expression.   Though this internal change may be miniscule, it can nevertheless be a powerful transformation that an audience often senses.   In an instant, what seemed to be an insignificant internal change can astonishingly captivate an audience. It is at this instant that the expressive power of internal change to communicate outwardly is perfected. This discipline evolved to be of utmost importance for a Noh actor.

'CONCEPT OF YUGEN' DEFINED AS THE EXPRESSION OF INTERNAL

This transformation is brought to life based on training of the performer, and is not acting in a generally understood sense. I think this transformation is a type of Yugen in Noh drama. That is to say, a Noh actor physical goal is to develop the body to be an artistic life form that can command internal change at will.   Having accomplished this, it is possible for all motions on stage to become an expression of Yugen.   Conversely, amateurs are incapable of imitating even the simplest gesture of a Noh master because although they may be able to mime what is visible, they are unable to alter phase of the body caused by deliberate mental control. Furthermore, this experience of the Yugen is not something brought about by relativistic stage production found in modern drama.   No amount of staging to alter the relationship between performer and audience will manifest this Yugen.   The Yugen is an expression of internal transformation that is consciously triggered in each performance. Once this physical development is attained, the body becomes an ecriture – a complete form of expression. The Kamae (posture) establishing a motionless stance by erasing all signs of breathing. An accomplished Noh actor breathing is different from an ordinary person.   When we say a masterful performer breathes naturally, we are not referring to every day, unencumbered respiration.   Rather we are referring to he breath of nature" grasped through long years of asceticism.   And the master is capable of using this naturalness to conjure an atmosphere at a blink of an eye.   The basic stance of Noh, the Kamae, is simply standing motionless on stage. And yet the actor must concoct an air of excitement and the feeling of tension with this simple

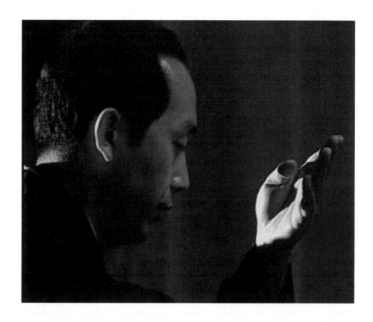

stance. The Kamae requires skill to immediately create a specific atmosphere without premise.

I think shape and form are unrelated to Kamae, and that the stance involves using the body to produce a specific ambience. Put extremely, I could be lying down on stage and still accomplish Kamae.

Breathing for the sake of conveying internal change outward in many cases is without sound, that is to say it is done in silence. This requires a sort of paradox, the desire to erase all signs of breathing. The anticipation of outward expression and an internal drive to stanch any sense of being must coexist in the body. For example, breathing can neutralize attitude, which is working internally on the performer body, so that this attitude is not projected outward. I repeat, what ought to be projected outward is the expression of internal transformation, and not the attitude of a performer. Unfortunately, in a bad way, audiences are usually more acutely cognizant of attitude than a performer is aware. When Zeami (1363 ? 1443), one of the founders of Noh, said ucceeding to hide is to bloom," I think he partially meant it as a admonishment against performers and their attitude.

A BODY THAT CAN EXPRESS THE MOON AND DEEP VALLEY

An actor has failed if an audience can sense what he is thinking in the back of his head. Ideally, only an image portrayal should be visible. In a poker game, often an opponent can succeed in reading your hand. This is an example of ones weakness being unconsciously revealed through ones facial expression. Failure of art occurs in this same unconscious sense. When I was small, I experienced a performance of Yamanba where the main actor performed a certain gesture up stage at the dramatic climax that whereby summoned a vision of deep valleys in front of my very eyes.   And when the main actor in Tohru sang he moon in particular has risen," I felt the moon exist inside my body.   These are good examples, in which image portrayal was successful.

The big problem with modern performing arts is that it often exhibits elements best remain unseen and fails to portray what ought to be visible.   We are appalled when we witness acting that is full of narcissism for no reason other than the actorattitude.   What the audience sees is a display of self-indulgence, not a physical portrayal.   In addition to experiencing the occult in the relativism of modern drama, we Noh actors strive for another aspect, to let the body itself begin talking as a means of expression.